PHYSIOTHERAPY ASSESSMENT

Physiotherapy Assessment

SECOND EDITION

ANNE PARRY, PhD, MCSP, DipTP
Senior Lecturer, Physiotherapy

with contributions from
NORMA BROOK, BSc (Hons), MCSP, DipTP
Principal Lecturer, Physiotherapy
and
CYNTHIA FOX, PhD, MEd, MSc
Senior Lecturer, Psychology

Department of Health Studies, Sheffield City Polytechnic

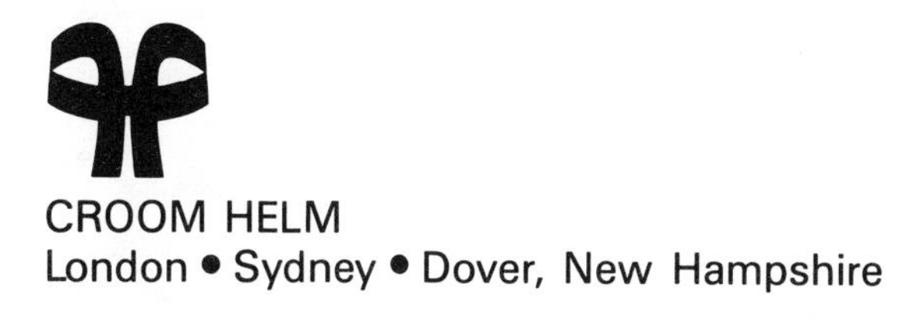
CROOM HELM
London • Sydney • Dover, New Hampshire

Croom Helm Ltd, Provident House, Burrell Row,
Beckenham, Kent BR3 1AT

Croom Helm Australia Pty Ltd, First Floor,
139 King Street, Sydney, NSW 2001, Australia

British Library Cataloguing in Publication Data

Parry, Anne, *1943-*
Physiotherapy assessment. — 2nd ed.
1. Physical therapy
I. Title II. Brook, Norma III. Fox, Cynthia
615.8'2 RM701

ISBN 0-7099-4009-2

Croom Helm, 51 Washington Street, Dover,
New Hampshire 03820, USA

Library of Congress Cataloging in Publication Data

Parry, Anne.
Bibliography: p.
includes index.
1. Physical therapy. 2. patient monitoring.
I. Brook, Norma. II. Fox, Cynthia. III. Title.
(DNLM: 1. Patient care planing. 2. Physical
therapy. WB 460 (P264P)
RM701.P37 1985 616.07'5 85-4615
ISBN 0-7099-4009-2 (pbk)

Filmset by Mayhew Typesetting, Bristol, UK
Printed and bound in Great Britain by
Biddles Ltd, Guildford and King's Lynn

CONTENTS

FIGURES

TABLES

ACKNOWLEDGEMENTS

Much of this book was written with knowledge gained through teaching students at Sheffield City Polytechnic and on clinical placements in physiotherapy departments in and around Sheffield. I am indebted in particular to Norma Brook for her contribution to 'Recording Assessment and Treatment' and for reading the typescript, and to Cynthia Fox for her contribution to 'Conducting the Subjective Examination'. I would also like to thank Julia McGuiness-Scott for the stave of Benesh Movement Notation in 'Recording Assessment and Treatment'; and Jan Connell and Liz James of the Physiotherapy Department, Northern General Hospital, Sheffield, for their patient attention and corrections to the descriptions of chest radiographs. I wish to acknowledge the collaboration of Carole Eales in producing the original versions of the 'Guides to Assessment' and the 'source-orientated record form' in 1976. Last but not least, special thanks are due to my colleagues who contributed to the first edition and to the students who offered suggestions for improving it!

Anne Parry

1 ASSESSMENT AND PRESCRIPTION

Nothing in this life is certain, except death and taxes — and change. The practice of physiotherapy is a vocation which is clearly changing from an occupation to a profession. It is implied by definitions in dictionaries that professionalism characterises a group of individuals whose practice is based on an organised body of knowledge, who train over a long period of time, and who belong to an association of peers which controls right of entry, maintains and enforces rules of conduct, and actively influences public policy in their field. The style and role of physiotherapists are subject to change too; and the pre-eminent concerns in physiotherapy today are different from the paramount concerns of twenty years ago. The changes of the last ninety years are more obvious, although some of the attitudes prevalent then are still detectable today. The medical press was publishing scandalous reports of objectionable and disreputable massage establishments when Rosalind Paget and Lucy Robinson conceived the Society of Trained Masseuses in 1894. One is reputed to have said to the other, 'A society of massage at this time — what will people think? What will the doctors say?' (Wickstead, 1948).

Those Victorian ladies needed the approbation of the medical profession to enhance their credibility as practitioners. They did not envisage examination and assessment by physiotherapists as a basis for prescribing their own treatment, but made it a rule of conduct of their new society that no cases would be undertaken without doctors' orders (Bromley, 1983). Consequently, treatments tended to come into fashion and go out of fashion according to whether or not they were prescribed by doctors. When the Professions Supplementary to Medicine Act (1960) came into force in the UK seventy years later, 'supplementary' was an accurate description because physiotherapy was still a treatment which, like drugs or any other treatment, had to be prescribed by a doctor on the basis of his diagnosis. Physiotherapists were considered to be technicians who carried out prescriptions. They made precautionary tests, such as tests of thermal appreciation prior to treatment with heat, and some tests to monitor patients' progress, such as grading muscle power; but they did not assess their patients in order to prescribe treatment.

During the last twenty years, research and innovations in areas underlying physiotherapeutic techniques have provided physiotherapists with knowledge to develop new methods of treatment and appropriate skills.

Research has also enabled them to understand the effects of their treatment and to advise against or to indicate possible dangers in their use. Inevitably, the focus of diagnosis and treatment changed as they became more able to rationalise the selection of techniques of treatment appropriate to particular pathologies and problems. Physiotherapists became more orientated towards symptoms and dysfunctions of individual patients, such as pain, limitation of the range of movement of a joint, weakness of muscles and poor co-ordination of movement. They became more concerned with evaluation of their treatment of individuals against the background of the person's life as a whole: and strongly prescriptive referrals by doctors became inappropriate.

Today, students of physiotherapy might laugh a little derisively at the idea of massage of the abdomen being prescribed for relief of constipation: but its efficacy has not yet been evaluated in a clinical trial. The quantity of research by physiotherapists has increased during the last ten years, and its quality has improved, in response to the important and fundamental changes in the philosophy, tactics and techniques of the practice of physiotherapy. These changes in practice require critical assessment of the patient, in order to establish priorities in dealing with symptoms, and critical appraisal of the effects of physiotherapeutic techniques and treatments, in order to select the most appropriate for each individual. In turn, this requires evaluation of the effectiveness of physiotherapy by physiotherapists. Ideas about the effectiveness of many techniques seem to be based currently on intuition: physiotherapists get a 'feel for things' through experience melded with instinct and subjective judgement based on insight. In order to test this intuition, the validity and reliability of procedures and measurements used in assessment need to be thoroughly tested first.

The first edition of this book was a response to the new syllabus and examinations by which the Chartered Society of Physiotherapy confirmed that, after referral, it is the professional responsibility of physiotherapists to ensure that patients are treated safely and effectively. In order to do so, physiotherapists should assess their patients and make their own decisions about treatment. Paradoxically, although professions develop through accentuating their distinctiveness, uniqueness and separate knowledge, development leads to closer, more integrated connections with allied professions. For example, ideas about the conduct and environment of assessments have become clarified as links with behavioural scientists have developed.

Physiotherapists' acquisition of a prescriptive role can be seen as a developmental stage in the process of maturation of physiotherapy as a profession which is allied and complementary, rather than supplementary, to medicine. Like every other profession, it is faced with the need to review its purpose in terms of changed circumstances, and to be active in bringing about desirable changes. Physiotherapists do not practise in a vacuum but face to face with members of the community they serve. Consequently, the profession must embrace knowledge, skills and techniques which enhance practitioners' capacity to employ new knowledge in order to solve specific problems of individuals and groups and to modify their practice in response to the needs of society.

The *Concise Oxford Dictionary* defines the noun 'need' in relation to circumstances and the verb 'to need' in relation to necessity and obligation. In descriptions of patient care, definitions of need have usually eluded the precision grip of those who have attempted to define it; and some of the qualities Macbeth ascribed to the dagger have been attributed to need (Acheson and Hall, 1976). Perhaps it may be 'the false creation of his oppressed brain', but there are no standard criteria of need or eligibility for physiotherapy and rehabilitation. The availability of services varies between localities and the level of provision determines accessibility (DHSS, 1972). Consequently, the limited financial income of the National Health Service is under pressure to redress inequalities in the provision of care as well as to accommodate extensions of all aspects of the service.

Although physiotherapists have added prescriptive and managerial roles to their traditional curative, restorative and ameliorative roles, the current situation is not ideal for totally effective care. The conflict involves knowing what ought to be done for individuals and the constraints imposed by the availability of resources, including physiotherapists' skills and the settings in which the skills are used. Conflict arises over the ordering of priorities although practitioners, planners and policy makers are all concerned with the two dimensions of provision of care described by Cochrane (1972): effectiveness and efficiency, or the ability of a procedure to alter the natural history of a condition for the better and the more complex issue of the ratio of the effect achieved to the resources used.

Physiotherapists are clarifying their notion of clinical autonomy. This must include strategies for dealing with the potential conflict in the relationships between the professions defined in Health Circular HC(77)33 (NHS, 1977): the referring doctor's right to retain overall control of the patient and to demand a certain treatment and the physiotherapist's right to refuse to carry out that treatment. Williams (1983) has pointed out that physiotherapists have a legal responsibility under their insurance cover to assess every patient and to assure themselves that proposed treatment is both appropriate and safe; and that to give ineffective treatment knowingly is a breach of professional responsibility to patients. A physiotherapist's right to refuse to carry out a particular treatment should depend on the findings of the assessment and her considered opinion both of the most appropriate treatment for the patient and of the safety or potential effectiveness of the treatment prescribed by the referring doctor. Consequently, physiotherapists have ethical, legal and professional responsibilities to ensure that they have adequate information in order to decide what is the most appropriate advice or treatment.

A miscellany of issues faces everyone engaged in health care. The concern is to arrive at solutions which will retain successful attributes, modify other aspects, and include entirely new concepts. The character and spirit of a profession are made real and operative through a dynamic process of refinement. For physiotherapists, the redefinition of their relationships with their patients is reflected in their assessment, a design for action which acknowledges uniquely physiotherapeutic responsibilities, provides a framework of approach to every patient the practitioner sees, and recognises the rights of patients in agreeing expectations for their own treatment. The prescriptive role requires assessment for physiotherapy to provide a vehicle for the formulation of aims of treatment and for evaluation of that treatment.

One of the most important implications of assessment for physiotherapy is that a physiotherapeutic interpretation, or 'diagnosis', is not the same as a medical diagnosis. In general, medical diagnoses are descriptive of disease processes, and one or two words are constellatory in that they imply what may take many pages of a text book to describe. Physiotherapeutic diagnoses are descriptive of the dysfunction of a particular system or part of the body, and they may change as treatment progresses and patients are reassessed. Two patients referred with the same medical diagnosis may not have the same physiotherapeutic diagnosis. For example, two patients are referred with osteoarthrosis of the knee joint. For one, the physiotherapist may decide that pain is the main disabling symptom; for the other, she may decide that limitation of joint range is paramount. Indeed, for a third, muscle weakness may be the main problem.

Additionally, although these patients may have identical detectable disease processes, the dysfunction experienced by any individual may be out of proportion to the describable signs and symptoms. Alternatively, some patients referred for physiotherapy may have no detectable disease process at all for which a medical diagnosis can be named: for example, patients complaining of low back pain. This does not diminish the importance of either the medical examination or the physiotherapeutic assessment. Rather, it emphasises the need to establish priorities in treatment in order to alleviate the symptoms and dysfunctions which are interfering with the person's life most.

There are three main steps to a physiotherapeutic assessment. To prevent confusion, the common practice of referring to the physiotherapist as 'she' and the patient as 'he' has been adopted.

(1) *Subjective examination:* listening to the patient's description of his illness and disability, how it has progressed, how it has interfered with his life-style, and what previous conditions might have precipitated or influenced it.
(2) *Objective examination:* collection of all relevant information through observing, palpating and testing.
(3) *Interpretation:* of the abnormalities of structure and function that were found during the examination and the psycho-social influences on function so that:
    (a) aims of treatment can be formulated which are compatible with the patient's goals and expectations;
    (b) means can be selected which are appropriate to the individual and are available within local constraints;
    (c) a programme of treatment can be planned.

The Subjective Examination

The aim of this examination is to determine the patient's symptoms, their distribution and behaviour, and how they are related to his health in general, to his social, occupational and domestic activities, and to his psychological well-being.

Although it is necessary to ascertain some basic information before embarking on the objective examination, history-taking is not a single event. It is a continuous process throughout assessment and treatment and the physiotherapist must be alert to important information which the patient may divulge during conversational asides while she is performing a test or treatment. Eventually, patients will be interrogated by a computer which can compile initial data more efficiently than a physiotherapist, but she will still have to listen effectively during assessment and treatment. Skills and techniques of interviewing are discussed in the following chapter.

Three types of history are important: the history of the present complaint; the social history; and the previous medical history. Although some of this information is available from the medical case notes, it is not a waste of time to ask the patient to repeat relevant reports. Firstly, it helps to establish a rapport with the patient; and secondly, the physiotherapist may ask questions in a different way to the doctor and receive additional or different information.

History of the Present Complaint

Except for patients with traumatic injuries, it is necessary to identify the complaint for which the patient first sought the advice of his family doctor, why he decided to seek help at this time, and what drugs he may be taking.

Firstly, a patient may describe symptoms which are not directly associated with the medical diagnosis but which may be his main problem, or confusing signs may be found on examination later. Additionally, patients commonly report a plethora of information, but the shape of the problem must be kept in sight: whether it is insidious and long-standing, or intermittent and long-standing, acute and improving, or acute and worsening.

Secondly, a traumatic social event, such as a bereavement in his family, may have caused him to seek attention rather than an exacerbation of symptoms. Similarly, people tend to date the onset of symptoms from a memorable social event; and questions about when the condition began should be followed up with questions about whether or not he had any problems before that event, or when he last felt completely free of the complaint.

The Social History

According to the type of occupation he has or the style of housing he lives in, a particular condition may render a patient temporarily or permanently unfit to work or to live at his home. Equally importantly for the individual, it may prevent him participating in a sport or another pastime. In order to formulate aims of treatment which are relevant to the individual, it is necessary to obtain a clear picture of his working and home environments and his recreational activities.

The Previous Medical History

This information is necessary in order to identify contraindicated methods and techniques of treatment. It is also necessary to know whether he has had physiotherapy previously, for what complaint and with what result.

The Objective Examination

The aim of this examination is to determine the degree of the patient's dysfunction through observing, palpating, measuring and testing, and comprehending results of tests recorded in the medical case notes. The examination should be ordered so that the patient is disturbed as little as possible and fatigued or exposed no more than is absolutely necessary. Signs which may be observed and palpated and tests which may be made are described in detail in the 'Objective Examinations'. The meaning of biochemical and other medical laboratory tests will be found in other text books and, except for a few which have particular significance for treatment, they are not repeated here.

In whatever order the examination is made, items should be recorded under main headings. 'Guides to Assessment' of patients with specific types of conditions are included in this book to direct students in particular. Recording assessments in this way will aid analysis of findings, show why particular interventive action was taken, and make it easier for another practitioner who reads them to comprehend them. The physiotherapeutic 'diagnosis', aims and selected methods of treatment should also be recorded.

Although physiotherapists seem to dislike keeping records, and to think that time spent on record-keeping would be better spent with their hands on patients, clear and concise records are essential so that a patient's progress through treatment is readily available. Additionally, comprehensive records of relevant findings and continuous notes on treatment and reassessment will aid writing of efficient short summaries for presentation at case conferences, on ward rounds, and for clinics they will allow continuity of treatment more easily if the patient is transferred to the care of another physiotherapist; and they will facilitate the retrieval of data for retrospective research or in case of legal enquiry. Various types of records are discussed in 'Recording Assessment and Treatment'.

Interpretation of the Findings

The object of the initial examination is to evaluate the patient's dysfunction in order to formulate aims which are pertinent to his needs and to plan a programme of treatment to fulfil them. Consequently, it is useful to review the findings with the following questions in mind:

> How much is this person's dysfunction related to his home, recreational or working conditions?

How much is his dysfunction related to psychological factors?
How much of his dysfunction can physiotherapy alleviate?

It cannot be said too often that there is no absolute value for 'normal' and a level of function which is acceptable for one person may be considered a disability by another person because of the different natures of their home conditions, their occupations and their life-styles in general.

Inevitably, some patients will be suffering from functional diseases, and they may be referred with the opinion that their symptoms have a psychosomatic origin. Physiotherapists' time is at a premium, to the extent that they must order their priorities in dealing with patients as well as with their symptoms. Therefore, a physiotherapist must decide whether it is within her role to treat these symptoms as real or whether she should discuss the patient's need for alternative help. Such a problem requires close liaison between clinical psychologists, doctors, physiotherapists and other practitioners. Some 'neuroses' appear to be partly physical and partly psychological, if only because a person in a state of anxiety cannot relax. Consequently, a person whose symptoms are a response to stress frequently derives benefit from physiotherapy. The hysterical patient rarely benefits unless behaviour modification underlies physiotherapeutic techniques because the (commonly paralysing) condition is the result of a subconscious conflict which usually needs the intervention of a skilled clinical psychologist, psychotherapist or psychiatrist.

Although it is difficult to prognosticate in many cases, it is necessary to consider how much benefit a patient can derive from physiotherapy. This judgement will determine the immediate and long-term aims and the means of achieving them. The prime need is to establish clearly specified goals which can be evaluated, these goals, which should be discussed with the patient, should be neither so high that they appear unattainable nor so low that they are not worth the effort. The decision about what is appropriate and achievable will depend on the knowledge, skill and experience of the physiotherapist.

When making these decisions, three related dimensions should be considered in relation to dysfunction and the individual patient's disability (see Figure 1.1). They are 'three distinct classifications each relating to a different plane of experience consequent upon disease' (WHO, 1980).

Firstly, the disturbance of normal psychological, physiological or anatomical structure or function causes *impairment*. Consequent interference with the person's ability to carry on his normal activities is *disability*. Thirdly, the disadvantage accruing to the individual from impairment and disability is *handicap*.

Figure 1.1: Dimensions of Disease and Disorder

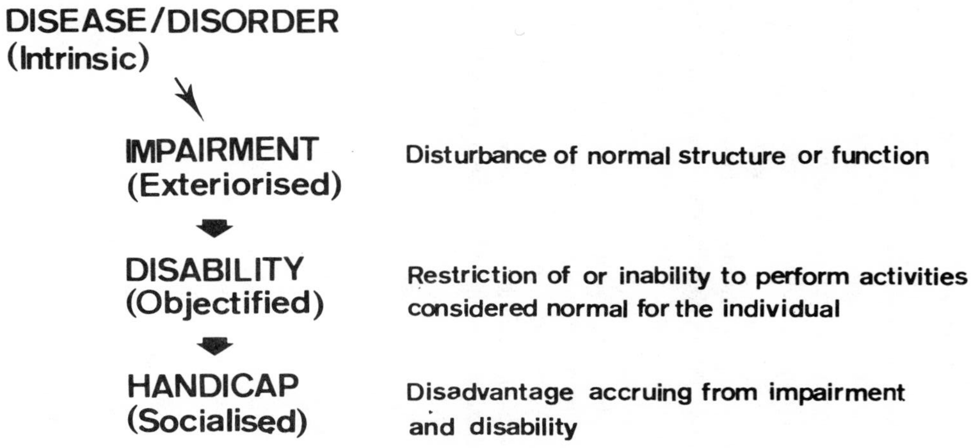

DISEASE/DISORDER
(Intrinsic)

IMPAIRMENT
(Exteriorised)

Disturbance of normal structure or function

DISABILITY
(Objectified)

Restriction of or inability to perform activities considered normal for the individual

HANDICAP
(Socialised)

Disadvantage accruing from impairment and disability

Therefore, the physiotherapist must consider not only her assessment of impairment and disability when formulating her aims of treatment but also the patient's perceived disadvantage, his individual social and psychological experience of disability, and his attitude towards his own incapacity. In discussion, realistic goals can be set which will make her aims compatible with his personal target.

This book is intended to introduce students to a systematic approach to assessment and to provide them with a guide to action, and to assist in the continuing education of those who were trained to fulfil the traditional role. Although those Victorian founder members might also be surprised at the extent to which physiotherapists' expertise has developed in particular clinical specialties, methods and techniques of treatment are beyond its scope. As it is concerned only with efficient and effective collection, recording and interpretation of information, it is expected that inexperienced physiotherapists as well as students will be able to discuss both the interpretation of their findings and the nature and duration of treatment itself with a physiotherapist who has appropriate knowledge and experience.

2 CONDUCTING THE SUBJECTIVE EXAMINATION

It may seem obvious to say that the function of communication is to convey correct meaning, except that every perceptive individual is aware how difficult it can be both to understand and comprehend what someone is trying to convey and to make themselves understandable and comprehensible. The view of social psychologists is probably most pertinent to physiotherapists: communication involves the totality of a person's behavioural and verbal responses (Argyle, 1972; Gagahan, 1975). Consequently, communication between a physiotherapist and a patient depends upon the way the physiotherapist touches the patient when she is palpating and making tests and the way she elicits information from him when she is taking the history.

Two considerations are fundamental to making the best use of the time available for interviewing a patient:

(1) How can the best and most informative history be gained which deals with the patient as a whole person?
(2) How can a knowledge of psychology help the physiotherapist to make sure that the interview is conducive to gaining a full understanding of the patient?

They require the physiotherapist to pay attention to setting the scene, at the bedside or in a treatment cubicle, to the pattern of her own behaviour during the interview, and to her interaction with the patient.

Interaction and Reaction

A skilled interview is essential if the patient is to enjoy optimum care, which includes good interaction with the carer. If the assessment is successful, patients feel that concern and understanding have been shown and they feel satisfied with the care given. Therefore, they are more likely to hold positive feelings towards the treatment which is prescribed for them.

For a variety of reasons due to prevailing conditions in wards and departments, a physiotherapist might not give sufficient thought to the environment and its effect on the patient when she is taking his history.

For example, the majority of patients have some degree of fear of things beyond their experience and, although the expectation of physiotherapy might not be the pain associated with dentistry, a cubicle full of electrical equipment will not calm their fears of the unknown. The physiotherapist may feel harassed and tired, but facial expressions which indicate anything but warmth and lack of eye contact with the patient are non-verbal messages which can ruin an interview. Argyle (1972) says that the non-verbal signals can deliver messages which are more potent than verbal communication — and the 'withering look' is well known! Additionally, by placing herself at a distance from the patient, the physiotherapist can indicate coldness and lack of real interest; and the way in which she orientates herself to him can signal many negative messages and can indicate that she is an authority figure who will make all of the decisions and who does not consider the patient a collaborator in his own treatment.

Many patients need to be given opportunities to express their fears and worries. This occurs after a rapport has been established during treatment usually, but it should begin during the assessment. Often, the history-taking revolves round the patient's physical condition; and decisions concerning future treatment which are based on this limited information can lead to a one-sided understanding of the patient. A successful history will permit assessment of a patient's problems in as many aspects of his life as possible, since only then can it be said that a comprehensive picture has been obtained. Indeed, in some cases the problems existing in the patient's environment are a greater feature in the presenting illness than are the physical aspects. Sometimes it is the patient's personality which is the major stumbling block since his attitudes to illness and his beliefs about his condition may be negative.

Therefore, it is of the utmost importance that psychosocial problems which may impede recovery are investigated. This puts an onus on the physiotherapist to be open-minded in her approach. Physiotherapists spend more time in fairly intimate one-to-one situations with patients than do most other practitioners; and, following comparatively brief and rushed consultations in general practitioners' surgeries and out-patient clinics, referral to a physiotherapist may be the first opportunity for them to reveal fears, worries and problems. Revelations may seem trivial or irrelevant to the physiotherapist, but they may be incapacitating the patient. A patient may want to admit drug dependence or suicidal thoughts, or to enquire about marital problems or sexual worries. The physiotherapist's reaction is vital. There should be willingness to discuss topics which need to be aired if full understanding is to be obtained. While it is not within the physiotherapist's province to tackle deep-seated problems, it is necessary for her to identify those which require referral to another professional or to give reassurance where it is appropriate. The quality of the therapeutic relationship throughout subsequent treatment may well be adversely affected if she shows embarrassment; if she is not aware of such euphemisms as 'my social life' or 'my married life'; if she chooses to ignore allusions or to reject a subject; if she has not thought out her feelings on such issues; or if she trivialises something which is of great importance to the patient.

Other mistakes in verbal communication also result in inadequate information being collected. The physiotherapist may dominate the talk or allow the patient to control the interview. Questioning may be badly handled — for example, too many closed questions might be asked and, although answers are gained, the right questions might not have been asked in the first place; or leading questions bias the interview in favour of the way in which the physiotherapist wants it to go; or several questions are asked at once without waiting for an answer to each one; or the patient may not be asked to clarify his comments or responses.

First Skills in Good Practice

The first necessity is awareness of the dangers of social perceptions. When meeting a patient for the first time, the physiotherapist reads cues which she uses to form a first impression of him. Such cues may be appearance, colour of skin, manner of speech and accent, name, address, type of illness, non-verbal signals, possessions: all of which help her to form a perception of the patient. Stereotypes are formed from positive and negative perceptions, and stereotyping can affect attitudes and behaviour. A positive perception augurs well for the interaction but, unless the physiotherapist is mature enough to hide her feelings, a negative perception may affect her attitude and behaviour to the extent that assessment and subsequent treatment are marred.

Furthermore, through the process of attribution, perceptions can initiate expectations which may bring about a 'self-fulfilling prophecy'. Attribution can lead to labelling, such as a 'well-motivated patient' or 'a no-hoper' or a 'won't-tryer'. For example, patients with chronic obstructive airways disease may either have a flushed face and puff or be cyanosed and bloated with oedema. Belcher and Sturridge (1972) say that 'pink puffers' can be regarded as 'doing their best' to keep down the level of carbon dioxide in the blood in the face of great difficulties; and that 'blue bloaters' have 'given up' and settled for poor levels of oxygen and carbon dioxide in the blood when they could 'try harder'. Labels like these influence practitioners' expectations of patients, and they stick.

Therefore, if on first meeting the physiotherapist perceives the patient as sensible and intelligent, she may attribute to him the qualities of common sense, reliability, understanding and high motivation even though these qualities may not have been exhibited. Consequently, she may expect him to be committed to treatment and to work hard; and he will probably oblige. Unfortunately, the converse also works, so that the physiotherapist can be a cause of unsuccessful treatment. Negative perceptions shared with other practitioners create more difficulties for the patient since he cannot avoid the consequences of labelling if he is referred to them.

It is best to try to ignore labels, to avoid taking expectations into the assessment, and to obtain further information before acting on initial impressions — and to remember that the process is two-way. The patient may already have expectations of physiotherapy and he will be forming perceptions of the physiotherapist throughout the assessment. If these are negative the physiotherapist will have to work hard to change them.

Stages in the Interview

(1) The first encounter should be warm and friendly so that the patient is able to feel comfortable and grow in trust. This can be achieved by ensuring that tone of voice, posture, facial expressions and orientation to the patient are cues which send messages of warmth and friendliness.

The chosen environment is also important in that many patients will feel inhibited if they do not have sufficient privacy. Curtains round a bed or across the front of a cubicle are inadequate if the patient feels that what is said is being shared by everyone else in the ward or department. The distance between the physiotherapist and the patient should be between two and three feet, since a shorter distance would be an infringement of personal territory and a greater one would be an unfriendly sign.

(2) It is important to find out the preferred name by which the patient likes to be addressed. In order to eliminate confusion on the patient's part, the physiotherapist should also indicate by what name she wishes to be called. It is sensible to talk for a while about general matters since this helps to set the patient at ease. Additionally, conversation can range freely and include topics which may have a bearing on his condition and treatment.

(3) Having put the patient at ease, it is important to explain the purpose of the interview. Illness and accidents leave their mark on patients and often affect their behaviour. Some become withdrawn, some become aggressive, and some give a picture of outward heartiness which is merely a defence mechanism. Whatever pattern of behaviour is revealed, the physiotherapist should make it obvious that she is accepting the patient with unconditional positive regard.

(4) The patient should be allowed to explain in his own words about his illness, his life and his attitudes. He is likely to have problems of a psychosocial nature associated with his physical impairment; so, if he does not disclose the full position but mainly talks about physical characteristics, enquiries can be made, such as 'How is the injury affecting your work?' and 'This situation must be difficult for your wife/husband/children.' In order to achieve such an open discussion, the physiotherapist will have to use questioning and listening skills effectively. While the patient is talking, she should engage eye contact to indicate attention to what is being said.

(5) Until computers are in universal use, history-taking should not be a stereotyped routine, even though answers to specific questions are needed. The physiotherapist must walk a thin line between conversation and formal consultation, directing the discussion by asking the patient to elaborate on points she considers important. Apparently straightforward statements may need clarification, such as 'What do you mean when you say that you do not feel well?' In particular, patients who use medical and pseudomedical jargon to describe their symptoms may not be using the terms correctly. Terms like rheumatism, slipped disc, angina or sprain should not be accepted without asking the patient to describe his symptoms. Concreteness may also be needed, such as when a recovering patient exclaims, 'I shall never walk again!' The physiotherapist can bring such a statement to a state of reality: 'You are having difficulty walking now but treatment will soon have you mobile again.'

(6) The patient's attitudes towards his condition should be identified. Does he exaggerate his illness or attempt to deny its existence? What does he feel about his future? Such detail gives the physiotherapist an insight into the patient's inner world. Both his illness and his attitudes and beliefs about it can affect his concept of himself. Whereas a positive self-concept can be helpful during treatment, a negative one can mitigate against success.

Apart from treating his physical condition, a physiotherapist will contribute to the patient's concept of himself by the way in which she fosters a positive body-image and deals with detrimental attitudes. It may be necessary for her to attempt to change his attitudes to create a climate that is more conducive towards treatment. Persuasion through communication and educating the patient about his condition are among the most effective methods of changing attitudes. However, change of attitude is not attempted lightly and can only be achieved if the patient is willing for the attitude to be changed. Also, the physiotherapist must examine her own motives and consider whether change of attitude is for the patient's benefit or for her own benefit.

(7) Finally, the patient will give clues about his personality while he is talking. He may be extroverted or introverted, but, whatever his personality, the physiotherapist has to assess the best way of addressing him in terms of her own behaviour. There is no pattern which embraces all patients and each individual needs a plan of action on the part of the professional which is unique to his psychological needs.

Conclusion

The interview should have unfolded and revealed a comprehensive picture of the patient's problems and needs. During the subsequent inspection and tests the physiotherapist can confirm her opinions or begin to explore issues not yet considered.

At the end of the assessment, she should explain what it will lead to in terms of treatment, explain any terminology, and give the patient time to ask more questions. For both of them, the work has only just begun. In discussion with the patient, problems have to be sorted into some sort of priority order and the methods of solving them considered. It may well be that no effective treatment of physical dysfunction can begin until psychological and social problems have been resolved, and that other expertise is needed. The point is that assessment of the patient as a whole has just begun and it must continue throughout the therapeutic relationship.

The session should also be terminated in the same spirit of warmth and friendliness which marked its beginning. The finale should be as positive as the introduction, and a handshake would not come amiss! The patient should have confidence in the knowledge not only that he is in capable hands but that the capable hands belong to a person who cares for the whole of his being and not just the part of his body affected by illness or injury.

3 THE OBJECTIVE EXAMINATION: INTRODUCTION

Skilful practice of physiotherapy is an art, not a science, but it calls on the tools of science in order to explain the phenomena of practice. Art concerns the ways and means of effecting certain outcomes, and scientific truth concerns fidelity to set standards. Consequently, while the objective examination requires skilful observation and handling, it also requires accurate measurement and verifiable results, so that the facts and causes of a patient's dysfunction are revealed, choice of treatment is based on sound judgement, and the effectiveness of treatment can be evaluated.

There is no short cut to efficient recognition of signs of disorder or to skill in making tests and interpreting results. Considerable guidance, training and practice are needed. In time, the skill becomes almost intuitive; but meticulous attention must be paid to the accuracy of procedures always. Spence (1953) described clinical observation as

> the craftsman's skill in seeing quickly what he knows to be significant . . . It is the product not of guessing but of sifted experience by which the significant is recognised with such rapidity that the steps of reasoning are not discernible to the uninitiated. (p. 629)

Consequently, the inexperienced physiotherapist must make her assessments methodically and with diligent attention to detail in order to add to her own knowledge, develop her skills of observation, and improve her ability to choose the most effective treatment. Ultimately, this will enhance the credibility of physiotherapy also.

The next four chapters of this book are a manual of procedures for assessment of the respiratory system, the cardiovascular system, the locomotor system and the nervous system. Every item in the assessment of a particular system may not be appropriate to the assessment of an individual with a condition affecting that system; and, whatever the primary condition for which a patient has been referred, it may be appropriate to include items of assessment of other systems. For example, a patient referred with an orthopaedic condition may need assessment and treatment of a chronic respiratory disease to enable him to undergo active rehabilitation.

Routines should be developed and applied rigidly and without variation so that nothing is forgotten. Examples of such routines are given in the 'Guides to Assessment' to assist students and inexperienced practitioners until they have developed their own preferred routines. Obviously, any routine will include examination of the part complained of and of possible sources of referred symptoms. A more general examination must not be omitted: it is necessary in order to form an opinion of the patient's general physical condition in relation to his psychological outlook indicated during the subjective examination.

The line between subjective and objective examination is not clear cut. In practice, the objective examination begins as soon as the patient is seen. The patient should be observed as he walks into the room, lies in bed or sits in a chair, and while he is talking. An overall impression is gained of his gait, his posture, and any gross deformities. Hands, ankles and feet can be very revealing, if not in relation to the first cause of his symptoms, then of factors which may influence treatment. The general state, shape and posture of a patient's hands may disclose information about his occupation and his way of life as well as his physical condition. Such signs as Heberden's nodes, trophic changes of the skin, tremor, clubbing, nicotine stains and calluses should all be noted. Swelling of the ankles and feet requires closer examination to determine the type of oedema.

Relief of pain is at the core of practice, but pain itself is a complex phenomenon. The expression in the patient's face and eyes should be observed. He may look ill or in pain; but it cannot be assumed that he is not ill or in pain because he does not appear to be suffering. Behaviour in illness (Zola, 1966) and pain (Zborowski, 1969) are said to be related to cultural background. Some people express their pain more than others do; and it has been shown that vocal patients receive more attention than quiet ones (Baer, Davitz and Lieb, 1970). The nature of pain of various types is presented throughout the assessments, and gestures indicating the character of pain are discussed at the beginning of Chapter 6. Difficulties may arise if there is a discrepancy between a patient's verbal account of pain and his gestures and other behaviour. He may say that he is not in pain when he appears to be so; or he may say that he is in pain when he does not appear to be. Physiotherapists must attempt to read all of the cues given by patients, bearing in mind its subjective nature:

> Pain is what the experiencing person says it is, existing when he says it does. (McCaffery, 1983)

All of the procedures in the following four chapters are laid out in accordance with a basic routine: (1) inspection: general and local observations;

(2) palpation; (3) specific tests and measurements. Unless it is otherwise stated, the part to be examined is exposed in a good light; and if one limb is being examined, the sound limb is exposed for comparison. A fourth part to the assessment of some systems presents medical data which may be obtained from the notes and taken into account when an assessment is interpreted and treatment is planned. Reference should be made to standard texts for descriptions of medical laboratory tests for specific conditions (see Evans, 1978). The assessor is expected to record nursing observations of the in-patient's temperature, pulse and respiration from his bed ticket and to count his pulse rate and rate of respiration for comparison during appropriate assessments.

4 OBJECTIVE EXAMINATION OF THE RESPIRATORY SYSTEM

Some patients are assessed in order to detect signs and symptoms which might predispose them to post-operative respiratory complications, some may be suffering an exacerbation of a chronic or long-standing condition, and some may have an acute infection. In each case, assessment of the respiratory system is directed at answering three questions:

(1) Can the patient ventilate his lungs effectively? That is, can he inspire sufficient air, is it distributed throughout all areas of the lung field, and is expiration unobstructed?
(2) Is adequate gaseous exchange occurring across the pulmonary membrane?
(3) What are the principal signs which will influence choice and application of treatment?

Physical manifestations depend on both the nature and the duration of a condition. Some variations are characteristic of particular conditions; and it may be appropriate to include items from the 'Objective Examination of the Cardiovascular System'. For example, it is necessary to assess the efficiency of the heart of patients with chronic obstructive respiratory conditions in whom there is a continuous spiral of cause and effect between the two systems.

INSPECTION

General Observations

Colour of Skin

Central cyanosis is a manifestation of the accumulation of reduced or unoxygenated haemoglobin due to inadequate oxygenation of the blood. It is apparent around the mouth: the tongue and the buccal mucosae appear blue but the extremities are warm.

Pink puffers. In the early stages of chronic obstructive airways disease

(COAD) patients attempt to compensate for changes in levels of blood gases by increasing their rate of respiration. The heart is induced to beat faster by the low tension of oxygen in the blood and the increased respiratory rate, resulting in a pink flush on the face. These patients breathe through pursed lips and dyspnoea may be intense but ventilatory drive is well preserved even if the airways are severely obstructed (Figure 4.1).

Blue bloaters. When the compensatory mechanisms are not effective patients become hypoxic and the right side of the heart fails increasingly. Consequently, there is visible central cyanosis and bloating oedema. Dyspnoea is relatively mild in these patients because they have poor respiratory drive. During infective exacerbations they expectorate large volumes of sputum and tend to drift into respiratory failure (Figure 4.1).

Effects of respiratory infection. Absorption of toxins will produce systemic effects such as loss of appetite, loss of weight and general malaise. Consequently, the patient may appear pale and emaciated. Additionally, respiration appears to be a great struggle and he is likely to look anxious because of the effort to oxygenate the blood adequately.

Local Observation

Shape of Chest

The thorax should be bilaterally symmetrical and narrower antero-posteriorly than from side to side. Postural deformities which affect ventilation may occur following thoracic surgery and as a result of chronic conditions.

Kyphosis is an increase in the antero-posterior curve of the spine. The shoulders are rounded and the normal lumbar lordosis is usually eliminated so the curve is a long one with its maximum convexity in the thoracic spine.

Scoliosis is a lateral curvature of the spine with rotation of the vertebral bodies towards the convexity. It may be a single curve in one direction only in one part of the spine, but there will usually be secondary compensatory curves.

Kyphoscoliosis is a combination of antero-posterior and lateral curves

Figure 4.1: Manifestations of Cardiorespiratory Insufficiency

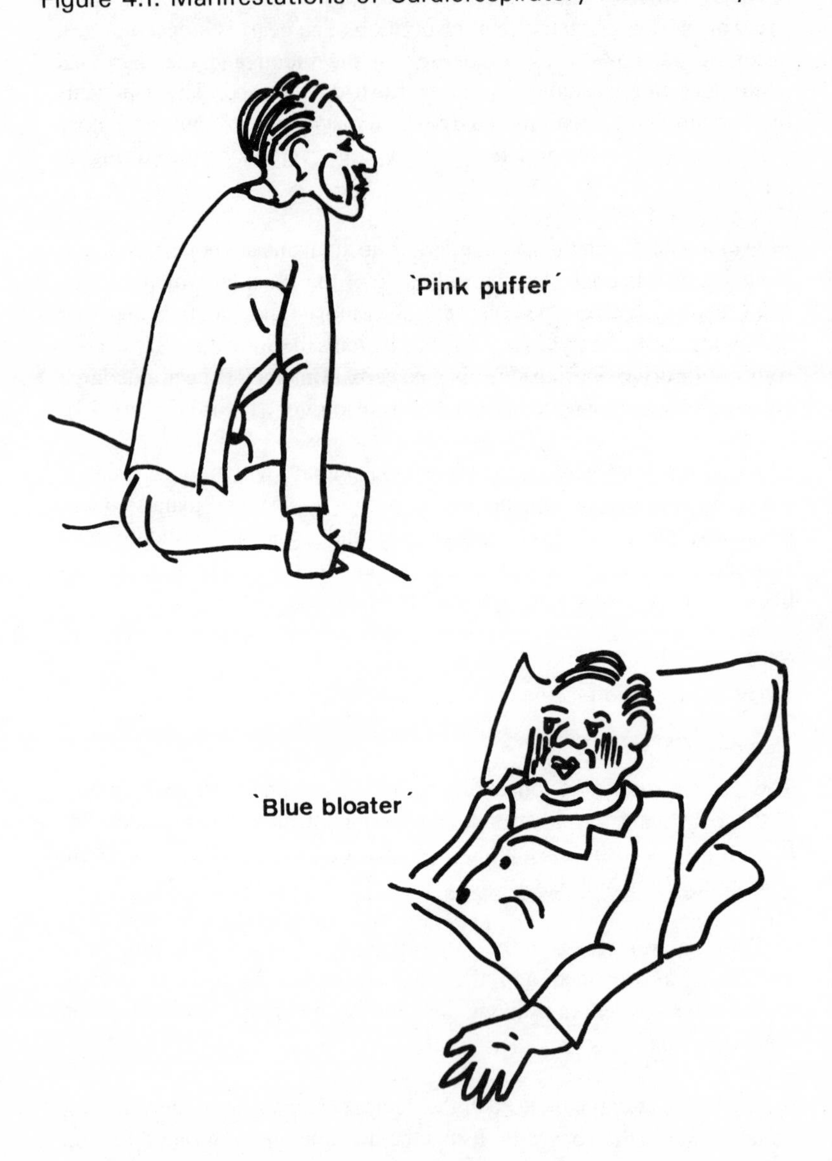

which is associated with ideopathic disorders of the vertebral column.

Long-standing respiratory disease causes pronounced alterations in the shape and mobility of the thorax, and specific diseases are associated with particular alterations in shape.

Barrel chest is a manifestation of obstructive airways disease, particularly emphysema and asthma. It describes dorsal kyphosis with increased antero-posterior diameter of the thoracic cage and deep sternal fossae. The neck appears short because the costal angle is decreased, the ribs are raised and more horizontal than normal, and the shoulders are high.

Funnel chest, or pectus excavatum, is a deformity of the sternum, costal cartilages and sternal ends of the ribs causing depression of the lower part of the thorax. It may be congenital and it is often associated with the development of kyphosis. Occasionally it is observed in asthmatic children due to the sternum being drawn in on inspiration.

Pigeon chest, or pectus carinatum, describes a very prominent sternum with an increase in the antero-posterior diameter of the thoracic cage. It may be congenital or acquired due to diseases such as rickets or chronic or recurrent upper respiratory tract infection in infancy. It is associated with the appearance of Harrison's sulcus, a transverse groove at the insertion of the diaphragm caused by deformity of softened ribs.

Rate and Pattern of Breathing

The resting rate of respiration of most normal adults is 12 to 15 breaths a minute. *Tachyopnoea* describes an increased resting rate which may be due to nervousness or disease.

Various aberrations may be seen and heard. For example:

(1) Inspiration may be prolonged in laryngeal and tracheal diseases.
(2) Expiration may be prolonged in bronchial and pulmonary conditions.
(3) Apical breathing is characteristic of chronic obstructive airways disease. Patients with chronic conditions attempt to increase the volume of the thorax using the accessory muscles of respiration. Consequently, the pectoral and sternocleidomastoid muscles stand out prominently, the rib cage rises and falls as a whole, and the abdominal muscles may work paradoxically during expiration.
(4) Children in respiratory distress may attempt to increase diaphragmatic excursion using strong contractions of the abdominal muscles.
(5) Patients with kyphosing conditions, such as ankylosing spondylitis, breathe diaphragmatically with little or no movement of the ribs.

Cough

Inspiratory noises are usually caused by obstruction of the larynx and larger airways, whereas expiratory noises are usually caused by obstruction of smaller bronchi and bronchioles. Following abdominal and thoracic surgery and through fear of pain or of bursting the stitches, patients may either suppress a cough or cough feebly and ineffectively. The type of cough will indicate to the physiotherapist which techniques of treatment are appropriate.

Short, painful, suppressed and unproductive coughing may indicate a medical condition, such as dry pleurisy, which cannot be improved by postural drainage. Post-operatively patients may adopt this pattern in order to inhibit coughing and avoid pain.

Loose, productive coughing indicates a condition, such as post-operative infections, bronchiectasis and lung abscess, in which ventilation and gaseous exchange can be improved by postural drainage.

Paroxysmal, ineffectual and exhausting coughing is a feature of asthma, chronic bronchitis and heart failure, and it may be aggravated by changes in the weather or temperature. It may need swift attention if it is accompanied by stridor, which can occur due to increasing tracheal obstruction following operations such as thyroidectomy or in children with whooping cough.

Nature and Quantity of Sputum

The presence of sputum is always abnormal, although many people consider it a natural phenomenon. Its quantity increases with the extent of pathological changes; its character will vary according to the presence or absence of bacteria; and its viscosity indicates ease of expectoration.

Mucoid sputum is scanty, clear, sticky and tough. It is caused by oversecretion of bronchial mucus produced by patients with acute or chronic bronchitis, bronchial asthma or the common cold.

Purulent sputum is copious, green or yellow, thick and foetid. It is caused by bacterial infection and produced by patients with post-operative infections, bronchiectasis or a lung abscess.

Muco-purulent sputum is caused by infection of the respiratory tract such as acute bronchitis.

Frothy sputum is copious, white or pink and aerated. It is a result of pulmonary oedema.

Haemoptysis

Fresh or old blood may be expectorated for a variety of reasons associated with vascular as well as respiratory conditions. Acute and chronic infections, inflammation of the respiratory tract, carcinoma, trauma, pulmonary disease associated with systemic conditions and occupational diseases such as pneumoconiosis may cause haemoptysis.

Rusty haemoptysis is old blood and its presence usually indicates resolving pneumonia.

Slight streaking of sputum indicates a bronchial lesion such as acute or chronic bronchitis.

Staining of sputum indicates mixing of sputum and blood peripherally in the respiratory tract, such as at the site of a lung abscess.

Frank haemoptysis is expectoration of whole blood which may occur with bronchiectasis, carcinoma, pulmonary infarction, mitral stenosis and tuberculosis.

Following thoracic surgery the sputum may contain frank blood which has seeped from the site of the operation. If haemoptysis persists postoperatively, or if any patient expectorates frank blood, respiratory physiotherapy should be terminated until the cause has been identified and dealt with. Haemoptysis of frank blood is potentially serious, and even small amounts expectorated during assessment or treatment must be recorded and reported.

Chest Pain

During assessment and treatment sometimes it is necessary to distinguish between pain caused by cardio-respiratory conditions and pain originating in other structures and organs. For example, hiatus hernia and ischaemia of cardiac muscle may be responsible for retrosternal pain and orthopaedic conditions may cause intercostal root pain. A physician must be consulted if there is doubt about the origin of any chest pain.

Central pain. Retrosternal pain which is made worse by coughing but not by deep breathing is usually due to inflammation of the trachea. Pain which is associated with dyspnoea, cyanosis and shock may be caused by pulmonary embolus.

Pectoral, axillary or dorsal pain. Sharp, stabbing pains which are made worse by attempts to breathe deeply indicate inflammation of the pleura with pain referred to the chest wall. Pleural pain may also be referred to the anterior wall of the abdomen. Severe, local stabbing pain with tenderness over the ribs may be caused by a strained intercostal muscle or a fractured rib due to trauma or metastases. Pleural 'rub' can be heard through a stethoscope and fractures will be apparent on radiographs.

Pain at the apex of either lung or over the anterior aspect of the shoulder. Sharp, stabbing pain which is made worse by deep breathing may be referred from inflamed diaphragmatic pleura or be caused by an abdominal condition. For example, flatulence under the left dome of the diaphragm can be referred to the left apex of the thorax.

Pain due to cardiac ischaemia is discussed in 'Objective Examination of the Cardiovascular System'.

Palpations

It is possible to estimate the extent and nature of movements of the thorax and the condition of the lungs themselves by placing the hands on the chest wall. When the chest is being palpated or measured the head must be supported to ensure that the accessory muscles of respiration are as relaxed as possible.

Localisation of Breathing

Hands are placed bilaterally over the main areas where movement occurs in order to compare expansion on both sides. That is, the hands are placed on either side of the manubrium sterni in order to assess the degree of apical movement, over the lateral aspects of the rib cage to assess lower costal movement, posteriorly below the scapula to assess posterior thoracic movement, and across the costal arch to assess movement of the diaphragm. Instruct the patient to breathe out, then to inspire fully and to breathe out again.

Expansion may not be bilaterally equal if a lobe or bronchopulmonary segment is consolidated or collapsed, in conditions such as pneumothorax, pleurisy with effusion, lobar pneumonia and tuberculosis; if expansion is restricted by fibrosis or neoplastic growth; or if movement is inhibited by pain due to a thoracic or high abdominal surgical incision or trauma such as a fractured rib.

Vibration

Vibration of secretions transmitted through the chest wall may be felt while localisation of breathing is being assessed. The exact location can be confirmed by auscultation and percussion.

Vocal fremitus. Distinct vibration should be felt when the patient is asked to repeat a number. Over some areas both hands will not feel vibrations of equal intensity because the heart diminishes fremitus on the left.

Increased fremitus indicates consolidation or a large cavity near the surface.

Decreased fremitus indicates bronchial obstruction or pleural effusion separating airways from the chest wall.

Percussion

The character of sound produced by percussion can be very informative. Normal resonance is altered when the normal air space in the lungs is obliterated. Place the middle finger of the left hand (if right handed) firmly on the part to be percussed. Flex the right wrist sharply and strike the back of the *middle* phalanx with the tip of the middle finger of the right hand.

Tap lightly and directly on the prominent points of each clavicle, then over each bronchopulmonary segment anteriorly on the right and left alternately. Repeat over bronchopulmonary segments laterally and posteriorly. Roll very ill patients from side to side in bed in order to tap their backs.

Normal resonance. The sound should be clear and low pitched, most resonant below the clavicles and scapulae and least resonant over the scapulae. Over the heart, the sound will not be equal to the sound at the same point on the right side.

Tympanic sound. This is increased resonance and indicates air in the pleural cavity, pneumothorax or a more or less collapsed lung.

Dull sound. This is diminished resonance due to consolidation, pleural effusion or pleural thickening.

TESTS AND MEASUREMENTS

Chest Measurements

These are a quantitative means of assessing movements of the thoracic cage. The normal range is very broad and, at the first assessment, a base line is established for the individual for comparison with measurements made serially throughout a course of treatment.

Measurements are made with a tape measure at three levels. Any three levels can be used as long as they are related to surface landmarks which can be accurately identified repeatedly. The commonly used ones are:

(1) at the level of axillae and sternal angle;
(2) at the level of the xiphoid process;
(3) at the level of the tenth costal cartilage or subcostally.

Support the patient in sitting with his arms by his sides and the accessory muscles of respiration as relaxed as possible, and instruct him clearly and fully before taking any measurements.

(1) Make resting measurements, taking care not to draw the tape tight as he breathes out.
(2) Ask the patient to breathe in fully. Do not record this measurement.
(3) Ask him to breathe out fully. Record the measurement.
(4) Ask him to breathe in again. Record the measurement.
(5) Calculate the difference between the two measurements and record the amount of expansion.
(6) Repeat this procedure three times at each level.
(7) Calculate the mean values at each level and make a permanent record.

Measurements should be recorded in a readily comprehensible format, as in Table 4.1.

If a patient shows paradoxical movement, which may result from severe emphysema, and measurement at the level of the tenth costal cartilage is greater on expiration than on inspiration, the difference should be recorded as expansion but preceded by a minus sign, e.g. $-\frac{3}{4}$ inch or -2 cm.

Auscultation

Comparison of breath sounds heard through a stethoscope on one side with those in the same location on the other side will support other observations concerning the free flow of air into and out of the lungs, bilateral

Table 4.1: Format for Recording Chest Measurements

MEASUREMENTS	AXILLA	XIPHOID PROCESS	10th COSTAL CARTILAGE
RESTING			
EXPIRATION			
INSPIRATION			
EXPANSION			

equality of breath sounds, and the degree of impairment of air entry on either or both sides.

In practice, use of the bell or the diaphragm of the chest piece is a matter of personal preference. In order to hear breath sounds clearly: (a) the patient must be relaxed and instructed to breathe through his mouth deeply and regularly but as quietly as possible; and (b) the chest piece must not be pressed against the skin or moved on it and the tubes must not touch any clothing.

Start to listen at the aspices where it is easier to hear breath sounds so that it will be easier to differentiate between normal and abnormal sounds at the bases. Work downwards, moving the chest piece from side to side, assessing at each point (a) the character of the breath sounds, and (b) the presence or absence of other sounds. Several kinds of breath sounds may be distinguished. There is some discrepancy in the use of terminology to describe them, and the conventions most widely accepted in the United Kingdom are used here.

Vesicular breath sounds are the normal noises which can be heard all over the chest wall over normal lung parenchyma. They are caused by turbulence in the air as it is deflected by the bends in the tracheo-bronchial tree. The inspiratory sound is a pronounced and easily heard rustle due to the air being drawn into narrower and narrower channels at a rapid rate of flow. It may be followed, without a pause, by the fainter expiratory sound which is about a third as long; but an expiratory sound may not be heard at all over normal lung tissues.

Collapse of alveoli decreases breath sounds and neither inspiratory nor expiratory sounds will be heard with complete atelectasis. They may be absent or very faint if a condition such as pneumothorax or pleural effusion prevents their transmission to the chest wall.

Bronchial breath sounds are high-pitched, brassy sounds which are heard over the trachea normally. Expiration is longer than inspiration and there is a short pause between them.

Loud and hard bronchial sounds will be heard during inspiration and expiration over an area of consolidation lying between a patent bronchus and the chest wall. There is a brief silence between the end of inspiration and the beginning of expiration but the sounds are of equal pitch, intensity and duration during each phase. They are of greater intensity than normal bronchial sounds because the air spaces are full of secretions.

Bronchovesicular breath sounds are coarse sounds which normally can be heard over the right apex, right interscapular area, main bronchi and the trachea. They may also be heard over areas of early consolidation, implying that some alveoli are still patent.

Adventitious (or added) breath sounds, known as rhonchi and crepitations, are heard over and above vesicular and bronchial breath sounds and indicate the state of the airways.

Rhonchi are sustained musical sounds of varying length and pitch which are usually heard on expiration and may be felt as vibrations through the chest wall. They are caused by the passage of air through airways which are partially obstructed by viscid secretions, bronchospasm, or oedematous mucosae. The pitch depends on the size of the lumen in which they are produced. Low-pitched sonorous sounds, such as the wheezing of patients with chronic bronchitis, are produced in the larger bronchi; and high-pitched sibilant or squeaky sounds are produced in small bronchi. Bronchospasm can cause both inspiratory and expiratory sounds. Inspiratory sounds which are due to secretions in the bronchi may disappear after coughing.

Crepitations are non-musical crackling sounds produced by fluid in the alveoli or smaller airways. They are most prominent at the end of inspiration and may also be heard at the beginning of expiration. If there is fluid in the alveoli, as in early pneumonic consolidation, fine crepitations or clicking sounds may be heard as the alveolar walls separate towards the end of inspiration. Coarse crepitations (called râles in some older texts) are produced by fluid secretions in the larger bronchi being drawn in with the air. They are characteristic of bronchiectasis and resolving pneumonia.

Pleural rub is a loud, dry, creaking, leathery sound which is diagnostic of pleurisy. It is heard in late inspiration and early expiration over the inflamed area.

Vocal resonance. The patient should be asked to speak while the stethoscope is applied to his chest. Normal lung tissue transmits booming low pitched frequencies and attenuates high frequencies. Consolidated tissue filters low frequencies and transmits higher frequencies so that speech sounds telephonic and bleating. Pleural effusion reduces the intensity of all frequencies. If he is asked to whisper, the words will be clearly heard through the stethoscope if the sound waves are conducted by consolidated tissue or a cavity communicating with the bronchus (whispering pectoriloquy).

Radiographs

Although radiologists' diagnostic reports of radiographs may be available in the notes, direct viewing of X-rays is essential to gain physiotherapeutically useful information. Additionally, in emergencies radiographs are returned to the ward before a radiologist has interpreted them and the physiotherapist on call should be able to make an immediate assessment. The radiograph is a two-dimensional picture of a three-dimensional object with one structure superimposed on another which creates certain problems of interpretation.

Routine chest X-rays (CXRs) of ambulant patients are taken postero-anteriorly (PA view) with the anterior wall of the thorax flattened against the plate and the arms internally rotated. Portable CXRs taken on the ward are taken antero-posteriorly with the plate behind the patient's back (AP view). Consequently, the heart and mediastinum appear magnified relative to the rib cage because they are further away from the plate than on a PA view. Therefore, serial PA views can be compared but PA and AP views cannot be compared with each other. A series of AP views may be compared if allowance is made for the fact that the patient's position in bed cannot be controlled exactly and, therefore, each CXR may be centred differently and the patient may be leaning further forwards or further back each time. Lateral views may also be available. The following points refer to examination of the straight coronal plate unless otherwise stated (see Figure 4.2).

(1) Identify the radiograph as a PA or an AP view. Usually it will be labelled. If it is not, the arms will be internally rotated on PA view and the scalpulae will be rotated so that their shadows do not obscure the lung fields.

(2) Decide whether or not the CXR has been centred accurately by

Figure 4.2: Chest Radiographs

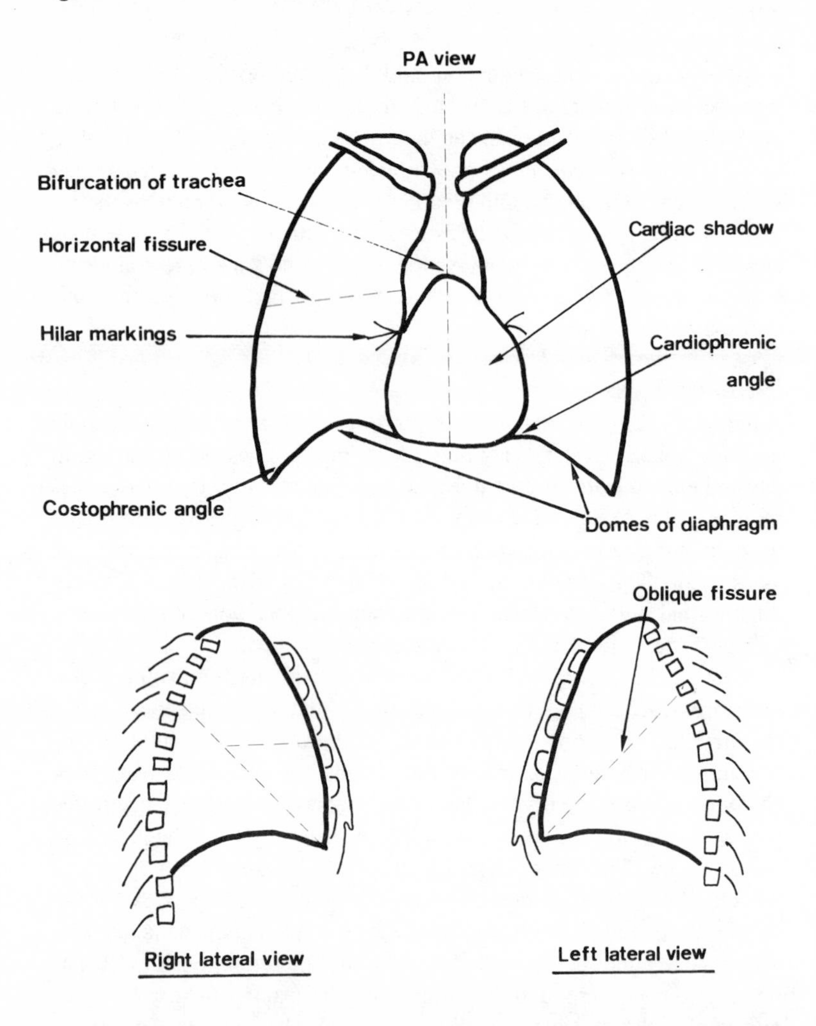

observing the symmetry of structures. The sternal ends of the clavicles should be equidistant from the midline or from the lateral edges of the vertebral body. The trachea should appear as a dark column of air centrally with the vertebral spines visible throughout its length. A slight bias to the right of the lower half of the trachea is normal. The hilar shadows may be slightly asymmetrical also: the vessels on the left may be 1 cm ($\frac{1}{2}$ inch) higher than those on the right and cast a less prominent shadow because they are partly obscured by the heart.

(3) Look at the outline of both domes of the diaphragm. The right dome should be higher than the left dome and the cardiophrenic and costophrenic angles should be acute and clearly defined.

(4) Look at the cardiac shadow. There is wide variation in its size, shape and disposition, but its position relative to the midline is fairly constant: one-third of its transverse diameter lies to the right of midline and two-thirds to the left. Apparent displacement of the cardiac shadow may be due to inaccurate centring. Earlier observations should have alerted the physiotherapist to the possibility of displacement resulting from scoliosis or deformities of the thoracic cage. Excluding these factors, the position of the cardiac shadow can help recognition of several conditions. (Observation of the cardiac shadow is discussed in more detail in 'Objective Examination of the Cardiovascular System'.)

(5) Identify the fissures of the lungs. Normally only the horizontal fissure is visible in PA view, and then in only 80 per cent of people. It should be level with the fourth costal cartilage anteriorly and the sixth rib posteriorly. In lateral view, the oblique fissures run diagonally downwards from the level of the body of the fourth thoracic vertebra and pass just below the tracheal bifurcation which is clearly visible. On the right it reaches the diaphragm 2.5 cm (1 inch) from the anterior costophrenic angle. It is more vertical on the left and reaches the diaphragm 4 cm (1.5 inches) from the anterior costophrenic angle.

(6) Examine the lung fields, working from apices to bases, comparing one side with the other. Normally ventilated areas are translucent.

Transparency of the lung fields is indicative of ventilatory efficiency. Recognition of abnormalities may assist selection of appropriate treatment and the most accurate and effective position for postural drainage.

Clearly defined opaque areas containing sputum or infected matter. Irregular pockets in the airways caused by bronchiectasis and large single shadows caused by abscesses can be accurately located prior to postural drainage.

Dense wedge-shaped opacities are caused by consolidated and collapsed areas. For example, collapsed left lower lobe will appear as a wedge in the shadow of the heart; and collapsed right upper lobe forms a wedge adjacent to the trachea. Resolution can be hastened by assisted coughing or postural drainage or both and re-expansion exercises.

Extrapulmonary dense areas may be caused by fluid in the pleural

Figure 4.3: Shadows Cast by Atelectasis

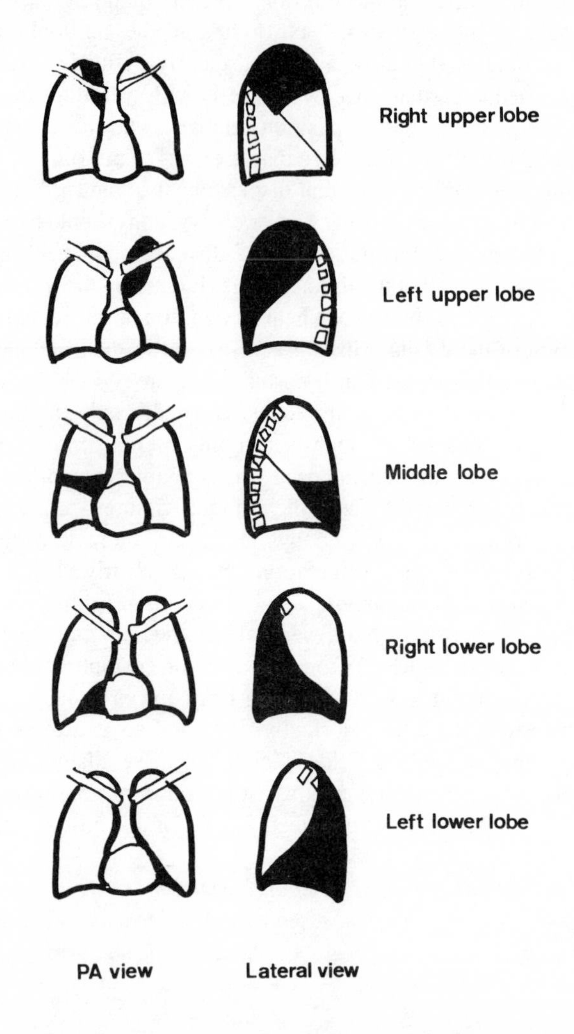

cavity. These cannot be resolved by postural drainage but breathing exercises are appropriate.

Hypertranslucence of both fields indicates over-distended alveoli such as are characteristic of emphysema. Re-education of breathing may be required. In asthma and emphysema, the diaphragm is abnormally low and the costophrenic angles may be obliterated.

It should not be forgotten that although physiotherapy is contraindicated for carcinoma, tuberculosis and pulmonary oedema, other medical considerations may outweigh the obvious contraindications.

Lobar atelectasis (Figure 4.3) is caused by obstruction of a bronchus by, for example, sputum, or a foreign body, or a neoplasm. Entry of air into lobules distal to the lesion and exit from them is obstructed, and air within the alveoli is gradually absorbed. An atelectatic lobe decreases in volume considerably, and this shrinkage is responsible for many radiological features. The diaphragm may be raised unilaterally and the trachea, the cardiac shadow and the visible fissures of the lung are displaced *towards the side of the atelectasis*. The rest of the lung appears more translucent and markings may appear to be diminished because unaffected lobes are over-distended. When all of the air is absorbed, the lobe becomes solid and casts a shadow on the radiograph.

Effusions of pus, blood or fluid into the pleural cavity cast a dense shadow and may displace mediastinal structures *to the opposite side*. Both the density of the shadow and the extent of displacement are proportional to the amount of fluid. Therefore, fluid may be more easily visible on a PA view than on a lateral radiograph, and vice versa. Effusion will gravitate to the lowest possible level in the thoracic cavity; and, if the patient is upright, a fluid level will be visible with an upward curve at the rib edge (fluid meniscus). Both the trachea and the cardiac shadow will be displaced to the opposite side and local flattening of the diaphragm may be apparent on the side of the effusion. After lobectomy fluid may collect in areas which the expanding residual lobe fails to fill. For example, after lower lobectomy it collects in the posterior costophrenic angle and after upper lobectomy it collects above and in front of the lower lobe.

Pneumothorax is caused by air leaking from the alveoli, the airways or the oesophagus. It may be seen as a hypertranslucent area with no lung markings, although the edge of the lung may be visible. As a general rule, physiotherapy is contraindicated for any patient with a pneumothorax. Spontaneous pneumothorax may resolve by absorption from the pleural space. Pneumothoraces caused by post-operative complications, such as a leak in the lung, bronchus or oesophagus or from a breakdown in the wound, may be associated with an effusion. Comparisons of the size of the shadow in serial films show if such complications are causing an increase in the volume of air. Occasionally, air accumulates rapidly, causing a massive pneumothorax and collapse.

Physiotherapy should be discontinued until a pleural drain is in situ and working.

Lung Function

The volume of air in the lungs and the volume of air which can be moved in one breath are related to physique and to the effects of respiratory disease. Various volumes can be recorded on a spirograph, as shown in Figure 4.4. Spirometry requires voluntary, sustained and maximal effort during inspiration and expiration for 15–30 seconds, which may be beyond the capability of some patients, it is likely to fatigue unduly many of those who can sustain the effort, and may produce bronchospasm in asthmatic patients.

Two types of machine are in common clinical use for measuring the capacity of the lungs and volumetric rate of flow of expired air. The Vitalograph records forced vital capacity if it is used statically and the forced expiratory spirogram if it is used dynamically. Lightweight, hand-held peak flow meters measure rate of flow of air. The basic technique is the same for each test.

(1) Ask the patient to remove or loosen any tight clothing which might restrict thoracic or abdominal mobility, such as collars and ties and corsetry.
(2) Let him rest for a while and explain the test to him.
(3) If he is taking the Vitalograph test, adjust the pedestal so that the tube is at the same height as his mouth in standing. Place a chair behind him so that he can sit down if he becomes dizzy or wishes to rest.
(4) Instruct him clearly about breathing in as deeply as possible before putting the mouthpiece in his mouth and breathing out. Demonstrate through a mouthpiece if necessary and allow him to practise through one. (Ask him to remove dentures if they prevent tight closure of the lips and might cause leakage of air.)
(5) When he is ready to take the test, allow him to hold the peak flow meter or the breathing tube of the Vitalograph machine, encourage him to breathe out maximally, take the deepest possible inspiration, and then blow out as hard as he can through the mouthpiece.
(6) Record his position accurately so that he sits or stands in the same anatomical position for any subsequent test.

There is considerable discussion at present about how many tests should be made and how the results should be used to calculate a value.

Figure 4.4: Static Lung Volumes

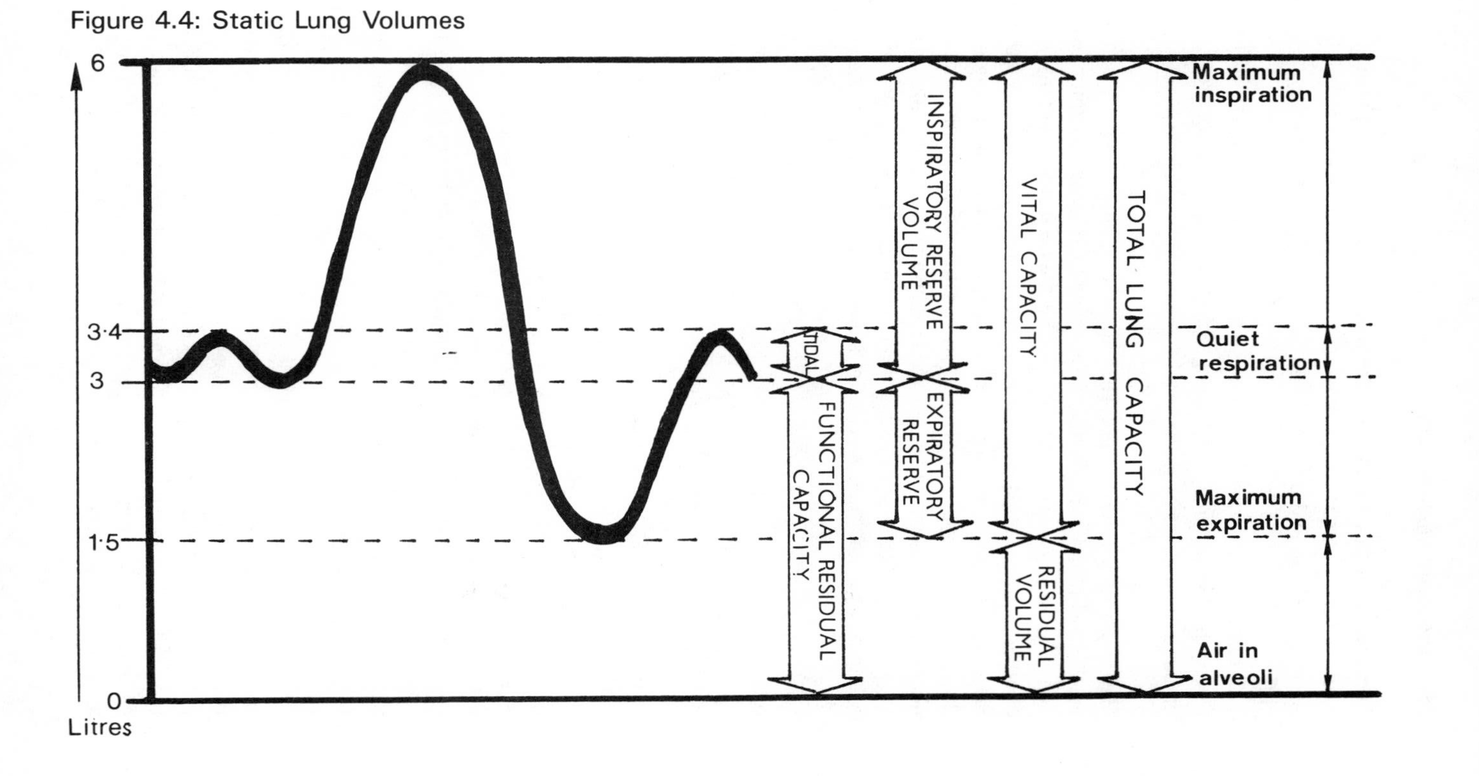

The assessor can consult both the literature supplied by the manufacturers of the machines and professional journals for more detailed discussion of rationale and interpretation. Commonly, vital capacity and rate of flow are measured three times and the values are averaged and recorded. The forced expiratory spirogram is recorded once, which will usually be the third breath into the Vitalograph machine including preliminary practice breaths.

Measurement of volume of air. The patient must blow into the Vitalograph machine as rapidly and as long as possible to achieve maximum expiration. The forced vital capacity (or FVC) is the measurement of the volume of air in a single breath which is indicative of the elastic properties of the lungs, airways and thorax. FVC varies with age and physique, but the minimum normal values are approximately 4.5 litres for men and 3.2 litres for women. The volume is reduced by any condition which reduces the elasticity of the lungs, such as fibrosis, or their capacity, such as lobar collapse, or both, such as consolidation.

Measurement of rate of flow of air. The forced expiratory spirogram records the rate at which the FVC is reached and allows the volume of air forcibly expired in the first second, or FEV_1, to be read. Normally, the FEV_1 is at least 75 per cent of the FVC.

Peak flow meters measure the maximal rate of flow during 10 milliseconds at the beginning of one forced expiration. The patient need not blow out to full expiration because the volume of air is not measured. The value obtained is called the peak expiratory flow rate or PEFR. Normal values for PEFR vary with age and physique also, but the normal range for men is 500–600 litres per minute or more and the normal range for women is 400–500 litres per minute or more.

Comparison of these values will indicate not only the most appropriate type of treatment, but how effective it is likely to be. For example, patients with emphysema may have restrictive and obstructive loss concurrently (Figure 4.5).

Restrictive loss. Both the volumetric capacity of the lungs and the volume of air which can be moved per breath will be reduced (a) if movements of the thorax are limited by deformities caused by conditions such as ankylosing spondylitis or kyphoscoliosis; or (b) if expansion and elastic recoil of the lungs are limited by conditions of the pleura or lungs such as fibrosis, pulmonary oedema and emphysema. For example, in long-standing chronic respiratory disorders where there is loss of compliance

Figure 4.5: Forced Expiratory Spirograms

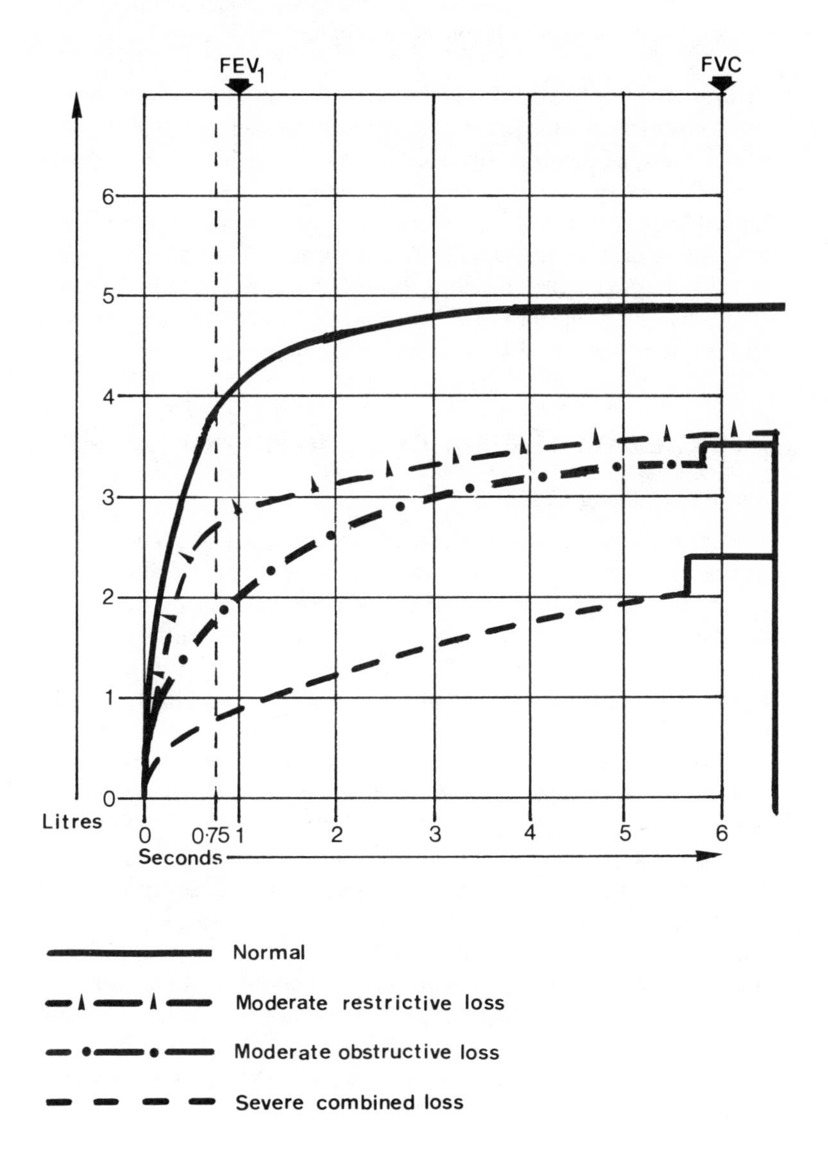

in the lungs, the FVC will be reduced because expansion is restricted and the FEV_1 will be less than 75 per cent of the reduced volume because the lungs are not able to recoil fast enough.

Obstructive loss. The PEFR and the FEV_1 indicate whether or not there is any obstruction to the flow of air. The obstruction is said to be reversible if both values improve following administration of a bronchodilating drug. This is likely with asthmatic and chronic bronchitic patients with bronchospasm. If there is no improvement, the obstruction is irreversible because there is structural damage, such as occurs with emphysema and chronic bronchitis. Therefore, a patient with chronic bronchitis may gain some improvement in PEFR from a bronchodilator but may still have some residual obstruction due to structural damage.

MEDICAL DATA OF SIGNIFICANCE TO PHYSIOTHERAPISTS

Analyses of Blood Gases

The partial pressure or tension of a gas is the quantity which determines its chemical and physiological actions. That is, the partial pressure of a gas in the blood determines its diffusion between alveoli and pulmonary capillaries or between tissues and systemic capillaries. Partial pressures of oxygen and carbon dioxide are calculated from specimens of arterial blood from the radial or femoral arteries and venous blood from the pulmonary artery or the right ventricle. Analyses of oxygen and carbon dioxide are expressed as PaO_2 and $PaCO_2$, where Pa denotes partial pressure in kiloPascals. Additionally, the concentration of hydrogen ions is expressed as pH.

In order to plan treatment it is necessary to understand the results of analyses which can reflect changes in functional adequacy of the lungs and perfusion of tissues before the effects are otherwise apparent. They may indicate a need for oxygen or suction or warmth, for change of position or adjustment of a respirator, or for deep breathing or effective coughing. The resting blood gases of 'pink puffers' are usually maintained within normal limits until they are terminally ill. 'Blue bloaters' tend to drift into respiratory failure with raised $PaCO_2$, hypoxia and heart failure.

Significance of PaO_2. The normal tension of oxygen in arterial blood ranges from 12–15 kPa (95–100 mm Hg). Patients with chronic respiratory conditions such as emphysema function with an arterial PaO_2 of 9.5 kPa

(70 mm Hg) or less. It is both unnecessary and undesirable to raise their PaO_2 to the normal level. However, it is desirable to raise the level of PaO_2 in patients who experience physiological shunting. That is, if patients are nursed in the same position constantly, some areas of the lungs will never be fully ventilated, some unoxygenated blood will be returned to the left atrium, and the PaO_2 will be lowered. Shunting will be diminished by changing the patient's position regularly. If his position cannot be changed, breathing exercises may improve ventilation and reduce physiologic shunting. Alternatively, oxygen may be administered at 40–60 per cent of inspired air in order to relieve symptoms, but without treating the cause.

The PaO_2 of venous blood may be less than the norm of 5.3 kPa (40 mm Hg) due to decreased cardiac output, haemorrhage with subsequent low volume of circulating blood, poor perfusion of the tissues causing peripheral vasoconstriction, and poor gaseous exchange in the lungs. In the last case, the patient may require administration of oxygen and suction to remove secretions.

Significance of $PaCO_2$. The normal tension of carbon dioxide in the blood ranges from 4.5 to 5.8 kPa (37–43 mm Hg). Raised $PaCO_2$ (hypercapnia) may result from increased metabolic rate due to fever or following surgery, or from retention of CO_2 due to pain. Retention of sputum following surgery or accompanying acute exacerbations of chronic bronchitis may induce respiratory failure: in which case it is necessary to clear sputum in order to increase alveolar ventilation and to encourage the patient to 'blow off' CO_2. If lung function is compromised by conditions such as emphysema it is not desirable to reduce ventilatory drive.

Significance of pH. The concentration of hydrogen ions determines the acid-base balance of the blood, with carbon dioxide on the acid side and bicarbonate on the base side. Normally blood is slightly alkaline. The arterial norm is 7.41 and the venous norm is 7.36, reflecting the rate at which CO_2 enters venous blood from actively metabolising tissues. Acidosis and alkalosis occur when the values fall below the norms and rise above them respectively.

5 OBJECTIVE EXAMINATION OF THE CARDIOVASCULAR SYSTEM

This chapter covers assessment of the efficiency of the heart and the competence of the peripheral vascular system. Many of the observations and procedures are appropriate to patients who are referred for treatment of conditions which affect other systems primarily. For example, patients with long-standing respiratory conditions are also likely to have some cardiac incompetence and surgical patients may suffer post-operative complications involving the peripheral circulation.

The principal manifestations of cardiac failure are due to compensatory mechanisms to cope with reduction in cardiac output and passive engorgement of vessels behind the failing heart. The heart may appear to fail as a whole but failure of the right side or the left side may be recognised in isolation in the early stages. Primary failure of the left ventricle occurs in coronary arteriosclerosis and when emptying of the left ventricle is resisted by aortic valvular disease or hypertension. Left-sided failure occurs secondary to mitral stenosis when the left atrium cannot empty blood into the left ventricle efficiently. The cardinal features of all forms of left-sided failure are lethargy due to the decreased supply of blood to the systemic circulation and dyspnoea due to congestion of the pulmonary circulation. Primary failure of the right side of the heart results from any condition which impedes emptying of the right ventricle; and it is associated in particular with emphysema and chronic bronchitis. Reduction of output of blood into the pulmonary circulation impedes venous return to the heart with consequent engorgement of systemic and portal systems. Oedema is the cardinal sign of right-sided failure. Frequently right ventricular failure occurs secondary to left-sided failure and signs of pulmonary congestion will already be evident.

The patient with a peripheral vascular condition may have a history which is typical of an occlusive condition, such as the limp caused by ischaemic pain in the calf muscles seen in Buerger's disease, or onset may be sudden, such as post-operative deep vein thrombosis.

INSPECTION

General Observations

Colour of Skin

Cyanosis is a bluish discoloration of the skin and mucosae caused by impaired gaseous exchange. *Central cyanosis*, which is evident around the mouth, is caused by imperfect oxygenation of the blood (see 'Objective Examination of the Respiratory System'). *Peripheral cyanosis* is due to oxygen depletion when the rate of flow of blood is slowed. It is visible as mottling of the skin of the extremities, particularly at the ends of the fingers and around the bases of the nails of the toes. It should not be confused with normal physiological responses to cold. *Pallor* of the skin of the lower limbs is a sign of occlusive vascular disease.

Oedema

Normal fluid balance is maintained by the relationship between the 'push' of hydrostatic pressure and the 'pull' of osmotic pressure of both the blood and the tissues. An increase in the circulating volume of blood is an important factor in the production of oedema in cardiac insufficiency, and its site is determined by which side of the heart is failing.

When the left side of the heart fails, a rise in pressure in the pulmonary circulation induces pulmonary oedema. The increased hydrostatic pressure of the blood overrides the osmotic 'pull' of the plasma proteins and water passes out of the capillaries into the alveoli. Chest physiotherapy is contraindicated in pulmonary oedema because it increases the stress on the heart and only serves to increase the pulmonary oedema. However, the need to clear the chest of infected pulmonary oedema may outweigh this consideration.

When the right side of the heart begins to fail, oedema results from reabsorption of sodium and retention of water by the kidneys. Consequently, not only is venous return to the heart impeded by right-sided failure but there is an increase in the circulating volume of blood: therefore, hydrostatic pressure is increased and the osmotic gradient is disturbed. The oedema may become generalised but usually it collects in dependent parts of the body; that is, in the sacral region if the patient is confined to bed and in loose tissues around the ankles if he is up and about.

Oedema of the lower limbs due to peripheral vascular inefficiency is indurated, or hard and organised. It is brought about by an effective reduction in osmotic pressure of the plasma proteins. In renal disease, oedema occurs because there is a real reduction in osmotic 'pull' due to reduction in the level of plasma proteins.

Some generalised oedema which resolves spontaneously is not uncommon in healthy women premenstrually. Localised oedema is seen in conditions which obstruct lymphatic or venous drainage, such as tumours, infestations, surgical excision of lymph nodes, and tight strapping or bandaging (see 'Objective Examination of Locomotor System').

Ischaemic Pain

Occlusion of arteries may cause several types of pain: a sudden agonising pain in the region of an obstructed vessel; a cramp-like muscular pain occurring during increased activity which is relieved by rest; or an aching or burning pain experienced at rest.

Cardiac ischaemia. Pain of relatively short duration associated with increased cardiac activity which is always relieved by rest is diagnostic of angina pectoris. The pattern is variable, but typically it is felt centrally and tends to spread across the shoulders and down the left arm. Myocardial infarction may cause a similar but more severe pain, feeling as if the chest is being constricted and crushed. Many patients do not suffer this characteristic pain, and some complain of referred symptoms such as indigestion.

Peripheral ischaemia. Vascular diseases which occlude arteries supplying the lower limb cause pain when the blood supply cannot cope with demands. Some patients complain of burning sensations in the limb when they are in bed at night. The blood supply is unable to cope with the demands of the skin as the limb warms up and the patient may prevent the discomfort by sleeping with the leg outside the bed covers.

Limping due to pain which is induced by exercise and relieved by rest is called *intermittent claudication*. Classically, while the patient is walking the muscles become ischaemic, he feels a severe pain in the calf and he limps, then rests to relieve it. The pain may be accompanied by parasthesia, such as pins and needles, more peripherally.

Local Observations

The Skin

The visible mottling of peripheral cyanosis may be apparent. Pallor is the more obvious sign of occlusive vascular disease and the skin may blanch visibly when the limb is elevated. The extremities feel cold to the touch also.

Circulatory conditions impair nutrition of the skin, which begins to atrophy, to lose hair and to look shiny and dry. Minor damage will be slow to heal and indolent ulcers may form, particularly in the lower leg. Pustular infections are common because resistance of the skin to infection is lowered. Gangrene is a complication of the later stages of peripheral arterial disease. A toe or another area of the foot may become blackened by dry gangrene or tissue destroyed by wet gangrene may slough.

Breathlessness

Breathlessness is a common feature of cardiac failure; but it should be remembered that people may be breathless for a variety of reasons, from nervousness to respiratory disease, which may be difficult to distinguish from underlying cardiac dysfunction in some circumstances. *Cardiac dyspnoea* is usually associated with exercise. The degree of cardiac failure can be estimated according to whether the patient is dyspnoeic on moderate exertion, on slight exertion, or at rest. Dyspnoea associated with effort is commonly abbreviated to *SOBOE*, meaning short of breath on effort. *Orthopnoea* describes distressing dyspnoea induced by lying. *Paroxysmal noctural dyspnoea* occurs when pulmonary congestion is induced by heart failure. The patient wakes up coughing ineffectually and paroxysmally and relieves the congestion by sitting with his legs dependent over the side of the bed.

Jugular Venous Pressure

Two or three small pulsations may be visible in the external jugular vein during each cardiac cycle (see Figure 5.1). They provide information about changes in pressure in the right atrium. The pressure of venous pulses falls during inspiration when blood is drawn into the heart and, in health, the mean height of the wave reaches the height of the manubrium sternum. Therefore, except for occasional visible pulsations, the jugular venous pulse, or JVP, is hidden below the clavicle whatever position the person is in. It may be visible if there is an increase in the circulating volume of blood, and a slight rise commonly occurs during pregnancy.

The mean height of the JVP can be estimated when the patient is half-lying with his head supported so that the muscles of the neck are relaxed. In mild right-sided heart failure, the pulse wave will be visible above the level of the clavicle while he is recumbent but not when he sits upright again. If pressure in the right atrium is very high, the height of wave

Figure 5.1: Raised Jugular Venous Pressure

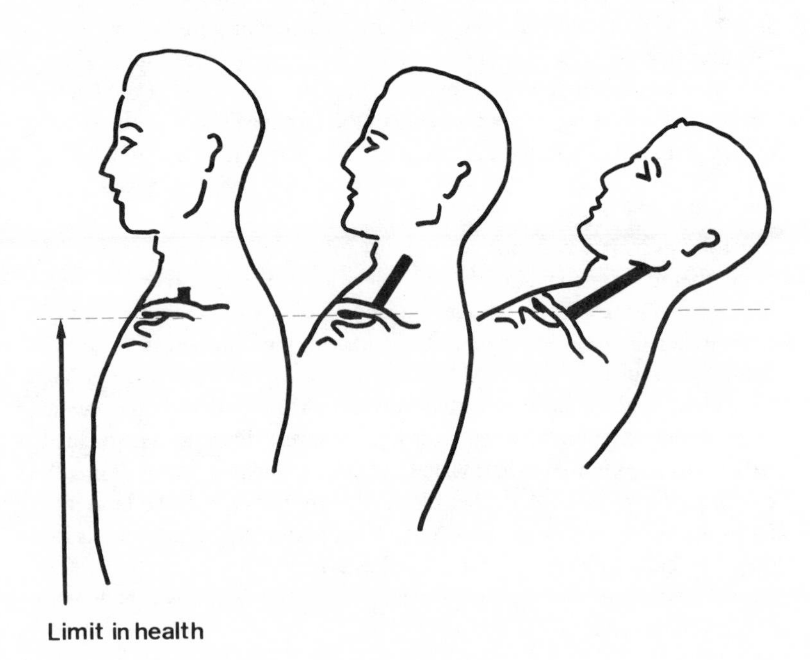

may be obscured behind the jaw when he is reclining and visible high in the neck when he is sitting upright.

Haemoptysis

Expectoration of blood is dealt with under 'Objective Examination of the Respiratory System'. Physiotherapists should be aware that haemoptysis may be a sign of cardiovascular conditions. For example, a patient with mitral stenosis may suffer profuse, and fatal, haemoptysis of frank blood due to rupture of dilated pulmonary vessels or of vessels under extreme pressure; or his sputum may be streaked with blood during attacks of dyspnoea; or he may expectorate pink, frothy sputum if he has pulmonary oedema.

Palpations

Apex Beat of Heart

As every candidate for the practical examination in Anatomy knows, the apex beat can be located in the fifth intercostal space on the left just medial to the mid-clavicular line with the person sitting or lying.

It may be displaced in a variety of conditions. Hypertrophy of the left ventricle displaces the apex beat to the left; and scoliosis and pulmonary conditions such as pneumothorax are responsible for displacement of the apex beat by displacing the heart as a whole.

Pulse Rate

Usually the radial artery is palpated at the wrist. The patient's forearm is pronated, his wrist is slightly flexed, and his pulse is palpated with the pads of the assessor's fingers. Time is allowed for quickening due to nervousness to subside before the pulse is counted for a full minute.

The normal resting pulse rate gradually drops from 120 beats per minute in childhood to 60–80 beats a minute in adulthood. The rate rises for pathological reasons such as shock, fever and thyrotoxicosis, as well as with exercise, nervousness and anxiety.

In order to increase their endurance, many middle- and long-distance runners aim to reduce their resting heart rate while increasing the volume pumped at each stroke so that the heart beats more slowly and more efficiently while they are running. Complete heart block may slow the ventricular rate to 20 or 30 beats per minute when the atria and ventricles beat independently because the impulse is not conducted through the atrioventricular bundle. In this case, the rate does not vary with exercise, the stroke volume is not increased, and the person may lose consciousness due to decreased cerebral blood flow.

Peripheral Pulses

The extent to which arterial disease is affecting the supply of blood to the lower limb can be estimated by palpating the femoral pulse in the femoral triangle, the popliteal pulse behind the knee joint, the anterior and posterior tibial pulses over the lower one-third of the tibia, and the dorsalis pedis pulse on the dorsum of the foot (Figure 5.2).

Pulses of both limbs should be palpated simultaneously and compared. The dorsalis pedis pulse may not be felt in the early stages of occlusive disease or if the occlusion is in the lower reaches of arteries. The palpable pulses will retreat up the limb as the blood supply is increasingly impeded. Findings should be compared with the reports of Doppler ultrasonic

Figure 5.2: Peripheral Pulses

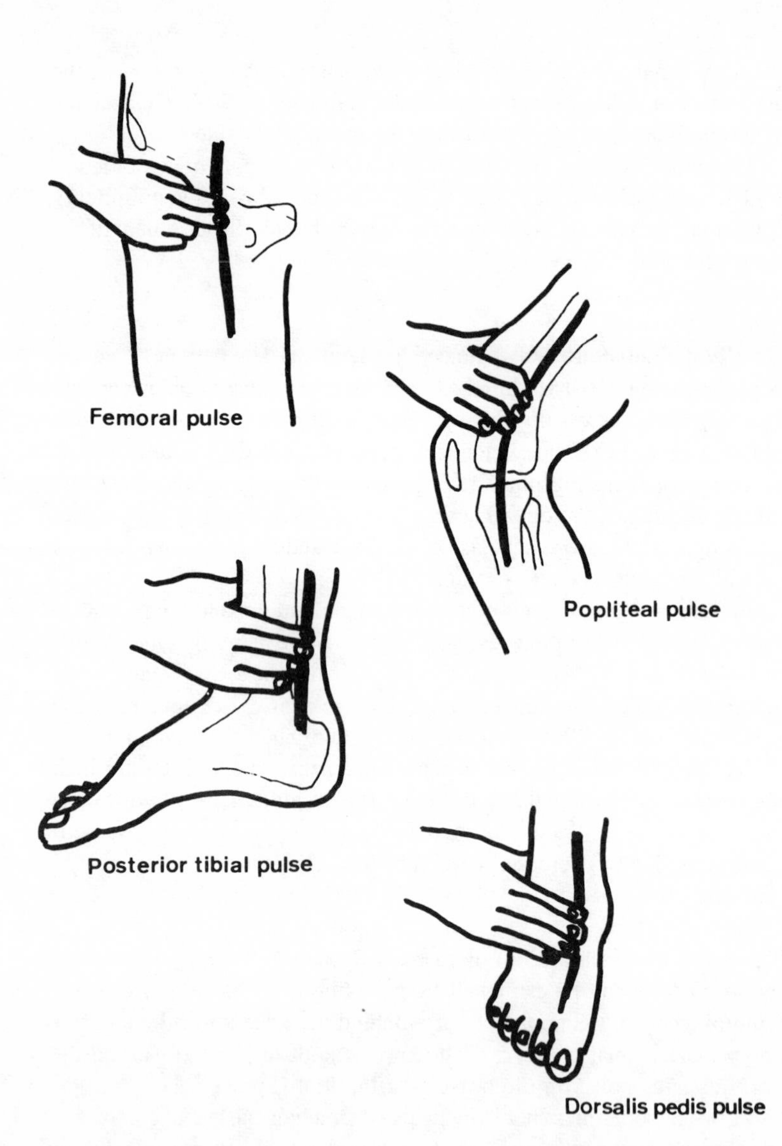

examination (see 'Medical Data of Significance to Physiotherapists', p. 55).

Homan's Sign

Thrombosis of the deep vessels of the calf is a potential and dangerous complication following surgery and for any patient who is confined to bed, particularly those on traction of the lower limb. The test for Homan's sign consists of passive dorsiflexion of the foot with the knee extended. Deep vein thrombosis (DVT) is indicated if pain is produced at any point along the course of the deep tibial veins. However, Homan's sign is an unreliable indicator because it is positive in the presence of less than 50 per cent of DVTs. The test should not be repeated because it can cause an embolus and subsequent pulmonary embolism.

More importantly, any complaint of tenderness due to pressure of the calf muscles as they rest on the bed or during maintenance exercises should alert the physiotherapist to the possibility of DVT. There may be some redness over the site of the pain, oedema and tenderness between the two heads of gastrocnemius. In which case it is unnecessary to test for Homan's sign: suspected DVT should be reported and exercise of the leg and foot must be terminated pending the outcome of more detailed examination.

TESTS AND MEASUREMENTS

Exercise Tolerance

Normally, the heart has considerable reserves and the limits are reached after considerable effort. As impairment progresses, breathlessness in particular becomes apparent with less exertion and then even at rest. Consequently, it is necessary to assess the heart's capacity for effort and any impairment of its reserve power.

Firstly, observe the effect of an everyday activity or an activity related to the patient's occupation: his colour, how much he sweats, how fatigued he is, and his emotional state. His functional capacity can be recorded using a classification such as that recommended by the New York Heart Association:

(1) Can withstand normal physical activity without provocation of symptoms.
(2) Symptoms develop only on moderate or severe exertion.
(3) Symptoms are progressive and are provoked by mild exercise.

(4) Cannot undertake any physical exertion without distress and symptoms may be present at rest.

Secondly, several indices can be recorded.

Respiratory rate. If the cardio-respiratory system can cope with the exercise easily, the resipiratory rate should be back to normal two minutes after it is finished.

Pulse ratio. There are several indices for estimating the capacity of the cardio-respiratory system for work. The simplest is:

(1) Take the patient's resting pulse for one minute before the exercise and record it.
(2) Take the patient's pulse at the end of two successive minutes after exercise and record.
(3) Add the two post-exercise counts together and divide the sum by the resting pulse.

The ratio does not exceed 2.5 for exercise that can be coped with easily. Several forms of exercise can be used.

(1) The Harvard step test, which is properly used with a more involved formula, requires the patient to step on and off a 30 cm (12 inch) high platform thirty times a minute for five minutes — or until he is unable to continue. This is a very severe test which is inappropriate for anyone with associated or secondary cardiac involvement.
(2) The standard step test requires the patient to step on and off a stool six times a minute for three minutes. This will be too strenuous for patients who become dyspnoeic during mild exertion such as walking up a slope.
(3) A daily activity such as getting out of bed, getting dressed, or rising from sitting in a chair can be used to make a functional assessment.

Walking rate. The distance ambulant patients can walk in a given time is recorded. The distance along level ground, such as a corridor, is measured accurately so that the full distance can be calculated from counting the number of lengths walked. Durations of six, ten and twelve minutes are suggested in various papers.

The patient is instructed to walk up and down as many times as possible and to rest as often as he wants but to stress himself so that by the end of the test he feels that he is unable to walk any further. He makes one practice walk the day before the test, or not less than twenty minutes before it. Although the test depends on the patient's motivation and willingness, it is said to produce usefully reproducible results.

Radiographs

Examination of radiographs of the chest is dealt with in greater detail under 'Objective Examination of the Respiratory System'. As interpretation of radiographs is an essential prerequisite to physiotherapy for respiratory conditions, it will be helpful if the physiotherapist can recognise some of the abnormalities associated with heart failure also.

The position of the heart in the chest, its size and shape and the outline of the aorta and the superior vena cava may be altered in disease. The normal cardiac shadow is shown in Figure 5.3 One-third should lie to the right of the midline and two-thirds to the left. Its transverse diameter should be no more than half as wide as the diameter of the lung fields. It may be enlarged by ventricular hypertrophy or dilation or by pericardial effusion.

The outline of the shadow should be looked at methodically:

(1) Look at the right border, at the outline of the ascending aorta and the right atrium.
(2) Look at the left border, at the outline of the aortic arch, the pulmonary artery, the left atrial appendage, and the left ventricle.

Left-sided heart failure, due to mitral stenosis for example, causes reduction of output to the systemic circulation and engorgement of the pulmonary circulation with consequent increase in pressure in the pulmonary artery.

(1) The aortic arch may be inconspicuous due to low cardiac output.
(2) The pulmonary artery is prominent due to increased pressure.
(3) The left atrial appendage is visible because the left atrium is enlarged.
(4) The lower left border is displaced because the left ventricle is dilated.
(5) Pulmonary oedema may be evident as patchy shadowing of the lung fields, as if they have been splattered with snowballs.

Right-sided heart failure due to emphysema or pulmonary fibrosis causes increased pressure in the pulmonary artery, because the pulmonary vascular bed is reduced, and leads to engorgement of the systemic circulation.

Figure 5.3: Normal Cardiac Shadow on Radiograph

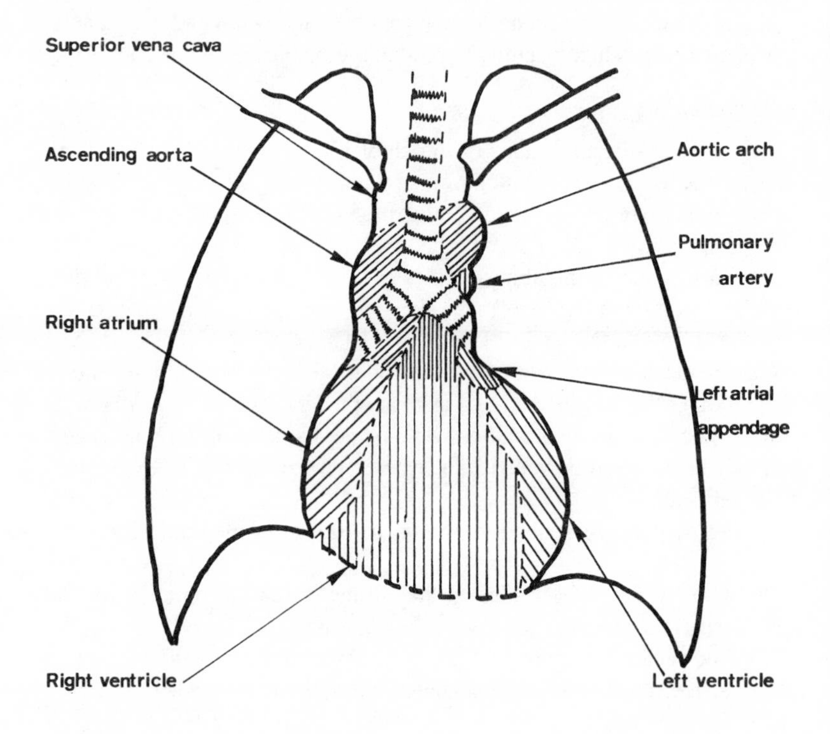

(1) The superior vena cava is dilated due to engorgement of the systemic circulation.
(2) The right atrium is prominent because it is enlarged or because it is displaced by the enlarged right ventricle.
(3) The pulmonary artery is prominent due to increased pressure.
(4) The left ventricle may be displaced by the enlarged right ventricle.
(5) Increased pulmonary vascular resistance may be evident as enlargement of proximal vessels with hypertıanslucence of peripheral lung fields due to reduction of the vascular bed.

Additional information which can help the physiotherapist to plan her treatment will be available from chest X-rays and reports of serial radiographs or high-speed cineangiography showing cardiac emptying of a contrast substance.

MEDICAL DATA OF SIGNIFICANCE TO PHYSIOTHERAPISTS

Arterial Blood Pressure

The physiotherapist may measure blood pressure with a sphygmomanometer before and after exercise or refer to the readings recorded on the patient's bed chart or in his notes. Although the technique is simple, results are subject to error by assessors. Consequently, discrepancies between reports on successive occasions, by the same and different assessors, may be due to assessors' inaccuracies rather than any true change in the patient's blood pressure.

The sphygmomanometer records both the pressure when the heart is contracting during its systolic phase and when it is relaxing during its diastolic phase. Blood pressure is still reported in millimetres of mercury rather than kiloPascals. In a healthy adult, the systolic pressure is equal to 100–140 mm Hg (13.5–18.5 kPa) and the diastolic pressure is equal to 60–90 mm Hg (8–12 kPa), reported, for example, as 120/90. The pulse pressure is the difference between the two pressures and should be no less than 30 mm Hg (4 kPa) and no more than 60 mm Hg (8 kPa).

In children, systolic and diastolic pressures should approximate to the lowest values for adults. It is not uncommon for elderly people to have systolic hypertension. That is, diastolic pressure is within normal limits but systolic pressure is raised because arterial walls have become inelastic. Very high systolic pressures are reached with arteriosclerosis; and low systolic pressures will be registered distal to an obstruction. Systolic pressures in the brachial artery and the posterior tibial artery are compared to detect arterial obstruction in the lower limb. An increase of more than 30 mm Hg (8 kPa) between a more proximal and a more distal segment of the limb indicates the level of the obstruction (see 'Doppler Ultrasonic Assessment', p. 55.

At all age levels, raised diastolic pressure is pathologically significant. It may occur secondary to renal or endocrine disorders, coarctation of the aorta or eclamptic or pre-eclamptic toxaemia of pregnancy. The cause is obscure in the commonest form, essential or ideopathic hypertension, which may result in hypertensive disease of the heart, cerebrovascular accident or deterioration of vision.

Auscultation

It requires a great deal of practice to be able to distinguish between the various sounds and murmurs produced in the heart and to focus on each event of the cardiac cycle in turn. Inexperienced physiotherapists may be able to hear only the two main sounds: 'Lubb', as the atrioventricular

Figure 5.4: Events in the Cardiac Cycle at 70 Beats per Minute

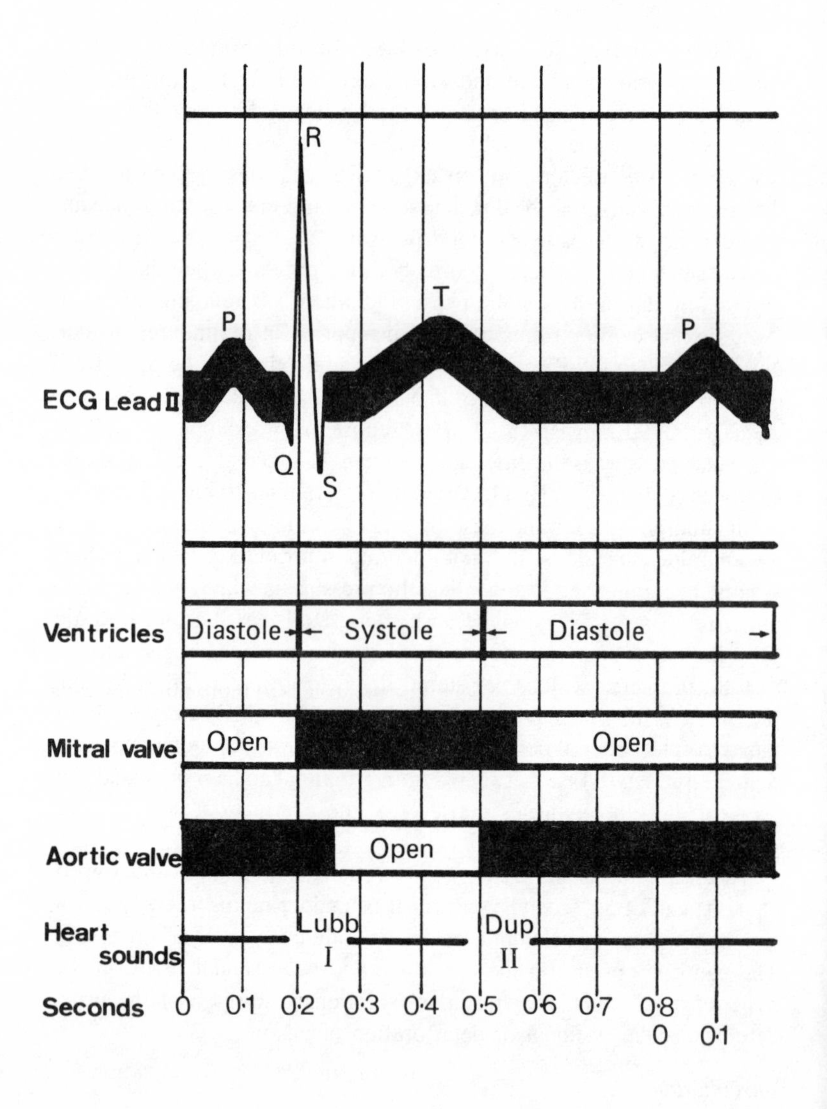

valves close, and 'Dup', as the aortic and tricuspid valves close (see Figure 5.4). Consequently, they should seek the advice and experience of a specialised physiotherapist or take information from the medical notes.

Electrocardiograms

The ECG records changes in electrical potential associated with contraction of the heart. Several different tracings can be obtained on graph paper by placing electrodes on the limbs or on different parts of the chest. Figure 5.4 shows the waves recorded from Lead II which is used for the bedside ECG. The waves are labelled P, Q, R, S and T. P is associated with the initiation of the impulse at the sino-atrial node and with depolarisation and contraction of the atria; Q, R and S are associated with depolarisation and contraction of the ventricles; and T is associated with ventricular repolarisation and recovery. Normally, the interval between the beginning of the P wave and the beginning of the QRS complex is less than 0.2 seconds and the duration of the QRS complex is less than 0.1 seconds. The whole cycle takes 0.8 seconds at 70 beats per minute.

ECG traces may show disorders of cardiac rhythm, ectopic beats, fibrillation of the atria or the ventricles, and heart block. For example, following myocardial infarction the ST segment is raised. Traces are analysed in relation to other clinical findings and considerable experience is required to interpret them accurately. Successive ECGs are made usually, and reports should be referred to regularly in case improvement is being indicated by restoration of abnormal traces to more normal waves.

Doppler Ultrasonic Assessment

The Doppler phenomenon is utilised to detect arterial disease, incompetence of venous valves, and obstruction of arteries and veins. An ultrasonic beam is directed transcutaneously at a blood vessel and blood cells in the path of the beam reflect an audible frequency. The change in the apparent frequency of the waves as a result of relative motion between the ultrasonic machine and the moving blood cells is analysed to determine the relative velocity of the flow of blood in major arteries and veins. The audible signals can be analysed to calculate numerical relationships between the frequencies reflected from different artieres and from different segments in the lower limb in order to detect differences in systolic blood pressure.

Angiography of Peripheral Vessels

Radiographs of vessels injected with a contrast medium disclose useful information about the patency of affected vessels.

6 OBJECTIVE EXAMINATION OF THE LOCOMOTOR SYSTEM

This chapter is concerned primarily with function of musculo-skeletal structures. Neurological disorders affecting locomotion are dealt with in 'Objective Examination of the Nervous System'. Many of these procedures are as appropriate to patients with dysfunction of traumatic origin, such as fracture of the shaft of femur, as they are to patients with conditions of more insidious onset, such as rheumatoid arthritis. Therefore, they are associated with several of the 'Guides to Assessment'. Some aspects of examination of the spine are also included, but no attempt has been made to describe the sort of detailed assessment which will be found in a specialised text on vertebral manipulation.

The aim of assessment of the locomotor system is to identify the manner in which a problem is manifesting itself and then to localise the source. The subjective examination will provide information about the site, nature and onset of current symptoms, their previous behaviour and details of any earlier treatment. The objective examination may demonstrate disturbances of function of the nervous system as well as the musculo-skeletal system if spinal roots are irritated or trapped.

Pain is the main complaint of many patients, and assessment of it may be inconclusive as far as localising a specific tissue or structure is concerned. However, the mode of onset may be significant in traumatic conditions; for example, although severe trauma may cause pain immediately, a forgotten injury may be responsible for an insidious pain which is becoming more persistent. Importantly, the patient's testimony regarding any change in the nature or distribution of pain is invaluable when the efficacy of treatment is evaluated. Before the objective examination is begun, the assessor should find out how the pain behaves at night, on rising in the morning, during daytime activities, and in the evening. She should also distinguish between constant pain with areas of radiation, periodic or episodic pain, and pain which is elicited or aggravated by particular postures or movement which can be examined later. She should watch the gestures he makes as he describes pain. He may indicate the character of the pain by making a clenched fist, by spreading his fingers widely, by alternately opening and closing his hand, or by jabbing with one finger. Additionally, he may keep his hand stationary on one part, rub an area, or point in a particular direction. Gestures like these may complement or conflict with words like 'severe', 'searing', 'burning' and 'stabbing'.

Local observations and palpations are described separately: in practice, examination of one part is usually completed before attention is transferred to another.

INSPECTION

General Observations

The patient's diagnosis, his medical notes and his description of problems will direct attention to specific areas. It is necessary to look for signs of muscle wasting, swelling and deformity more generally, and for rheumatoid nodules and outgrowths such as Heberden's nodes.

Gait

The opportunity should be taken to analyse the patient's gait as he walks into the treatment room or around the ward in his usual footwear. A truer picture is likely to be gained than when he knows that he is being watched when he has been asked to walk up and down. He should be observed walking barefoot also.

The pattern of gait may be disturbed by pain, stiffness of joints, impairment of muscle function and discrepancies in real and apparent length of limbs. Characteristic waddling makes the Trendelenburg gait easily recognisable. Other intrusions and interruptions in the pattern may be more difficult to identify. The rheumatoid patient, for example, may complain of 'walking on marbles' due to subluxation of the metatarsophalangeal joints, or may have 'foot drop' due to peripheral neuropathy, or show signs of spastic paraplegia if the cervical cord is compressed. The most obvious disturbance may be of cadence: that is, mistiming of rhythm and discrepancies in length of step. Analysis of gait involves several phases:

(1) general looking and listening for deviations from the normal reciprocal pattern;
(2) detailed observation of the swing phase and stance phase of both legs;
(3) interpretation of faults;
(4) identification of primary causes and secondary manifestations.

Additionally, he should be observed rising from a chair and sitting down again. In each case, the alignment of one segment on another should be judged at the first metatarsophalangeal joint, the ankle joint, the knee joint, the hip joint, the lumbar spine, the thoracic spine and the atlanto-occipital joint.

Posture

A variety of postures may be adopted by choice to relieve pain or to compensate for limitation of ROM in a particular joint. Metatarsalgia, for example, can have an effect on gait which becomes habitual, and the altered pattern of walking may result in increased stress at the hip and knee joints with consequent symptoms and signs. The curves of both the cervical and the lumbar spine may be altered to compensate for loss of extension in the thoracic spine, and the lumbar lordosis may be increased to compensate for restricted extension of the hip joint. The primary restriction must be identified and lost movement restored in order to avoid secondary stress of this type.

Specific points for observation are shown in Figure 6.1. A plumb line will make it easier to identify deviations. Discrepancies can be confirmed by tests for specific deformities. Patients with spinal conditions should be observed from all sides — sitting on a stool, standing, and flexing forwards in sitting and standing. If possible, they should be observed in prone and supine also.

Local Observations

Colour and Condition of Skin

Pallor or cyanosis indicates circulatory defects and conditions disturbing oxygen tension in the blood. Redness due to hyperaemia indicates an inflammatory reaction which might be local or systemic. Patients with rheumatoid arthritis look pale if they are anaemic, and they may have vasculitic lesions such as ulcers.

Contour and Alignment

Normality varies from person to person and the contours of the part on both sides should be compared, whether the disorder is unilateral or bilateral. No one is totally symmetrical; and undue prominence or localised changes in contour and attitude may be asymptomatic, or they may be the result of long-standing adaptive shortening, or they may indicate that free movement is hindered at some point in the normal range by acute

Figure 6.1: Observation of Static Posture

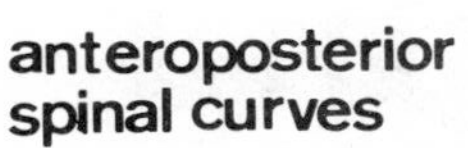
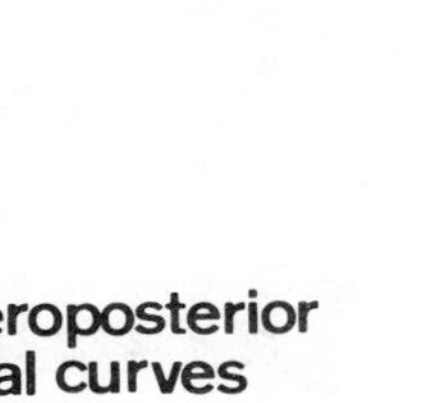
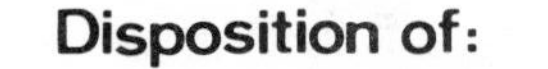
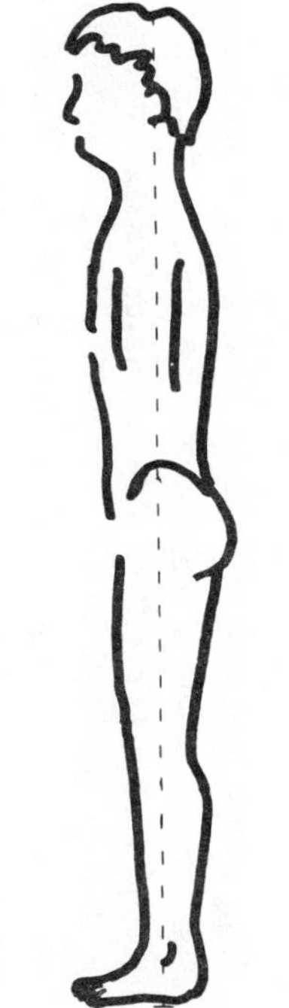
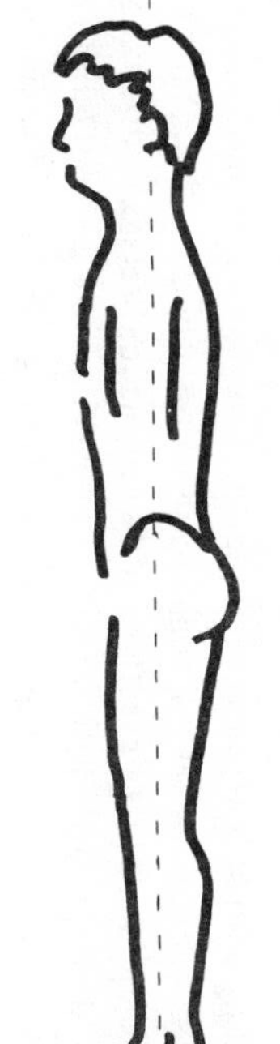

changes in soft tissues.

Localised swelling associated with injury is usually the result of trauma of capillaries and the release of histamine and related substances. Tight bandages, strapping or a plaster cast can cause oedema of a limb distally by obstructing venous and lymphatic drainage so that hydrostatic pressure is raised at the venuous end of the capillaries.

Effusion within a joint and swelling of soft tissues produce both increase in size and masking of subcutaneous anatomical detail. Atrophy of muscles decreases the curving form and outline of soft tissues and accentuates subcutaneous bony points. Misalignment of segments of the body may be caused by bony deformity and by alterations in muscle tone. Hypertonic muscles and their tendons which are subcutaneous will stand out prominently and flaccid muscles will hang away from the bone loosely. These alterations in muscle tone are dealt with in 'Objective Examination of the Nervous System'.

Deformities of Joints

A deformed joint is one which cannot be returned to the neutral anatomical position voluntarily. Bone or soft tissue or both can be responsible for obstruction or restriction. There is a wide variety of causes, for example:

(1) dislocation or subluxation due to congenital deformity, such as congenital dislocation of the hip or as a consequence of disease such as rheumatoid arthritis.
(2) imbalance of muscular pull resulting in dominant muscles and soft tissues contracting with a joint fixed in a particular position; for example, flexion-abduction deformity of the hip joint after amputation above the knee, and deformities due to paralysis and spasticity (see 'Objective Examination of the Nervous System').
(3) contracture of muscles and soft tissues as a result of injury or disease; for example, scarring of the skin after burns, Dupuytren's contracture of the palmar fascia, and Volkmann's ischaemic contracture of muscle.
(4) tying down of tendons in their sheaths; for example, flexion deformities of the fingers.
(5) postural and ideopathic deformities, such as the habitual adoption of a position due to pain and progressive scoliosis of unknown cause.

Conditions such as rheumatoid arthritis result in profound disruption of joints involving several mechanisms, which the swan neck deformities of the fingers and ulnar deviation of the wrists illustrate. However, the distribution of body weight is the determining factor in many acquired deformities. Consequently, many of the deformities of practical importance to physiotherapists are most apparent in the joints of the lower limb; for example, flexion-adduction of the hip joint in osteoarthritis and flexion deformity of the knee joint in rheumatoid arthritis and osteoarthritis.

Deformity of the hip joint is commonly due to pain on weight-bearing when the joint is in the close-packed position, with maximum tension of the capsule and ligaments. A position of flexion associated with adduction and lateral rotation is adopted to ease the joint. In time a fixed deformity may result from contracture of soft tissues, and the patient compensates for it by tilting his pelvis forwards and increasing his lumbar lordosis. If the hip joint becomes fixed in adduction, there will be an alteration in the relative positions of the lower limbs and the pelvis so that the transverse plane of the pelvis is not at right angles to the line of gravity.

Deformities of the knee joint may result from primary or secondary processes. Inflammatory processes in the knee joint are associated with effusion, a marked increase in intra-articular pressure, and severe pain. Semi-flexion of the knee joint, called Bonnet's position, enlarges the capacity of the knee joint, reducing pressure and relieving pain. Gradually, the bulk and power of the extensor muscles are reduced and the flexor muscles become dominant and shorten, producing a flexion contracture. Eventually, stress on the ligaments and capsule will produce organic changes with possible backwards subluxation of the tibia on the femur.

Changes in the alignment of the hip joint, ankle joint or the small joints of the foot may require the patient to flex his knees in order to stand upright. Maintenance of the flexed position is responsible for myogenic contracture with subsequent changes in the capsule and ligaments of the joint, and even in the bone. There is a direct relationship between the severity of flexion deformity of the hip joint and the degree of resulting deformity of the knee joint; and walking is possible only with great effort if the fixed loss of extension exceeds 40°.

Varus or valgus deformity of the knee joint may also be observed. Patients with joint disease associated with laxity of the collateral ligaments tend to bear more weight on one tibial condyle than on the other. This causes loss of height of the weight-bearing condyle eventually. Diminution of the lateral condyle causes valgus deformity or lateral angulation of the distal segment on the proximal segment: that is, genu valgum or knock knees when the tibia is so disposed to the femur. The pull of muscles, particularly tensor fascia latae, increases the deformity. Loss of height of the medial condyle causes varus deformity or medial angulation of the distal component: that is, genu varum or bow legs. Varus and valgus deformities may be ideopathic, or either may occur transiently in children when one femoral condyle has grown faster than the other. Up to 10° of valgus is said to be normal in women. Occasionally, valgus deformity of one joint and varus deformity of the other causes 'wind swept knees'.

Deformity due to fixed lateral rotation of the tibia on the femur occurs in about 50 per cent of moderately affected knees of patients with rheumatoid arthritis. It occurs in conjunction with valgus deformity and posterior subluxation of the tibia on the femur, which is associated with involvement of the talonavicular joint.

Deformities of the talocrural and subtalar joints. Varus-valgus deformities or contracture of the posterior tibial muscles and the tendo achilles will prevent the foot being plantigrade. Fixed dorsiflexion is rarely seen except in one of the congenital disorders which combine these deformities: congenital talipes equinovarus describes plantarflexion with medial angulation; and congenital talipes calcaneovalgus describes excessive dorsiflexion with lateral angulation.

Palpation

The patient may be anticipating pain, so warm the hands and allow them to rest for a moment on the limb to engender confidence. While it is necessary to find areas of undue tenderness of superficial bony points and soft tissues, it is neither necessary nor desirable to squeeze or to poke with the fingertips. Make firm but gentle movements to feel the contours of structures and to determine areas which give rise to pain or tenderness on pressure. At the same time, the temperature of the skin, its texture and excessive dryness or moistness, can be noted. It must not be forgotten that palpable asymmetry of contour and movement is not necessarily abnormal: such signs must be interpreted in relation to both the patient's reported symptoms and to other observations and tests.

Swelling of Soft Tissues and Joints

Swelling may be soft and fluctuant or thickened and indurated. Muscle bellies should be pliable and resilient, and muscles which are in spasm will feel unduly hard. Haematoma may be responsible for tense swelling in the belly of a muscle and inflammation due to trauma or disease may be responsible for swelling of soft tissues or joints. If enlargement of a joint is due to effusion into its cavity, fluctuation can often be elicited by placing one hand over the joint line and compressing the swelling from the opposite side. Bulging of the capsule will be felt under the palpating hand. A 'patella tap' may be heard from the knee joint if the effusion is gently squeezed from the patellar pouches with one hand and the patella itself is sharply tapped onto the femur with one finger of the other hand.

Thickening of Tissues

Localised thickening may be felt over the site of a painful lesion of a periarticular structure, even of joints which cannot be palpated directly, such as those of the spine. This type of thickening may be due to spasm of groups of fibres or of small intervertebral muscles, or it may be indurated oedema with some fibrotic thickening of the capsule or a ligament.

It is difficult to tell except by biopsy whether swelling of rheumatoid joints is due to effusion or to hypertrophy of the synovial membrane. However, enlargement due to thickening of periarticular structures feels fibrous (see 'Passive Movements', p. 64). Thickening by osteophytes in osteoarthrosis feels irregularly bony in contrast to the smooth contour of the periphery of subluxated joint surfaces. Bony tumours, callus and misalignment of malunited fractures may be felt on the shaft of a bone.

Pain and Tenderness

In the absence of other signs and symptoms, tenderness does not necessarily indicate abnormality. Some bony prominences are naturally tender, and some people are particularly tender over the clavicle or the processes of the thoracic spine.

When a tender area is discovered, it is necessary to determine its extent and to localise it as accurately as possible. Tenderness around a joint may arise from within the joint or in neighbouring structures. It may be necessary to provoke pain in order to confirm which structure is giving rise to it. For example, the patient may be required to perform a provocative exercise to simulate the situation in which pain is induced; or pressure with a flat hand on a spinal segment may provoke guarding spasm locally; or a test of the integrity and stability of a joint may cause pain.

Temperature

A part which looks red will also feel hotter to the touch than surrounding skin. However, where inflammation is subcutaneous the part may feel warmer than the same part contralaterally or another normal area without appearing red. Conversely, a decrease in temperature implies reduction in circulation, which can occur when a part is not used normally.

Tonicity of Muscles

The degree of resting tone varies from muscle to muscle and comparison with the contralateral muscle is essential. Both decreased tone and spasm of isolated muscles or groups of muscles are associated with pain in a joint or soft tissues.

Localised Passive and Accessory Movements

Joints are moved passively through full range, or as full range as is available, in order to feel the nature of resistance during the movement and at the end of the movement. Palpation of accessory movements must not be overlooked either, because any restriction can limit range of movement, impair the function of joints under stress and affect the patient's functional ability.

Passive movements. Before joints are moved passively the active range of movement must be estimated so that the assessor does not attempt to stress the joint beyond the available range. When a peripheral joint is being assessed:

(1) the patient should be asked to move the contralateral sound joint through its full range first of all so that the assessor can observe it.
(2) the assessor should move the sound joint through full range passively, so that the patient knows exactly what he is expected to do with the affected joint when it is being palpated.

Normally, there is no resistance during the movement; full range is reached when tissues are at the limit of tension; and there is detectable elastic resistance when slight overpressure is applied. Some people have hypermobile joints, which is of no consequence if it is asymptomatic. Abnormalities of various types may be felt:

(1) resistance felt during the movement may be due to guarding spasm or it may be voluntary.
(2) no resistance to movement but restriction of range with a hard feel to the end of the movement suggests bony limitation such as contact between the articular surface and osteophytes.
(3) a rubbery resistance during the movement of restricted range or rubbery rebound on overpressure at limit of restricted range suggests fibrosis.

(4) a 'boggy' hypermobility with no real feeling of end to the movement suggests serious pathology which requires reference back to the consultant.

Accessory movements. It is necessary to assess the extent of any increase or restriction in the range of accessory movements. They may be limited by thickening of connective tissue causing moderately painful restriction of movement, guarding spasm due to pain, or localised spasm at the beginning of the range due to irritability of nerve roots. Palpation of antero-posterior gliding, such as that which is available between the proximal and distal rows of the carpus, may demonstrate that free range of movement is limited due to restriction of accessory movements. Increase in their range may be painful or painless and may arouse suspicions of instability, such as occurs in the knee joint due to laxity of cruciate and collateral ligaments (see 'Tests: Integrity and Stability of Joints', p. 73).

Adventitious Sensations

While the joints are being moved passively with one hand they should be palpated with the other hand. A torn meniscus in the knee joint may produce a clicking sensation. More commonly, a grating or creaking sensation known as crepitus may be felt, and it may be audible. Although crepitations are usually found in osteoarthrotic joints, they are found in apparently sound joints also. They are usually more evident during active movement and, although the patient may report them, they may not be felt at all while the joint is being moved passively.

TESTS AND MEASUREMENTS

Muscle Strength

Except where an isolated muscle is affected, assessment of functional groups of muscles is adequate for most conditions affecting the locomotor system. The standardised method proposed by the Medical Research Council, which is also known as Oxford grading, is the most frequently used test. It examines the ability of a muscle or a group of muscles to perform a simple movement *through full range*. The starting position is chosen carefully so that trick movements are obviated and strength can be graded accurately on the following scale:

0 = no contraction
1 = flicker or trace of contraction
2 = active movement with gravity counterbalanced
3 = active movement against gravity
4 = active movement against gravity and a stated resistance
5 = normal functional power

Unless muscles are so obviously weak that only a flicker of movement is likely to be produced, testing at grade 3 is a useful starting point. If the patient cannot contract the muscle or group at grade 3, he is tested at grade 2. Alternatively, if he can contract at grade 3, he can be tested at grade 4. It should not be forgotten that 'normal' is a subjective value for the individual and it must be judged in the light of the individual's occupation and usual activities. With unilateral lesions of the limbs, the strength of muscles of both limbs can be compared, taking handedness into account when the upper limb is being assessed.

Some clinicians feel a need to record a value for muscles which can produce some movement but not through full range, or a value between grade 1 and grade 2 for muscles which can produce full range movement if they are assisted by gravity but not if gravity is counterbalanced. It is better to make a written note than to qualify grades with plus and minus signs which introduce more subjectivity and may cause another clinician to misinterpret the results at a later date.

Muscle Bulk

It is impossible to measure the bulk of any single muscle or any one group of muscles. However, comparison of circumferential measurements and volumetric displacements can be used to assess atrophy and swelling.

Circumferential measurements. Some idea of the shape of the limb and loss of bulk or increase in mass can be obtained by making measurements at varying distances along the limb from a suitable bony landmark. With the limb fully supported and the muscles relaxed, measurements are made to three or four points on the limb, including the region of most apparent atrophy or greatest girth. The skin is marked at each point and the distances from the bony landmark to them are recorded. The limb is encircled with a tape measure at each point, taking care with the position of the tape on the underside of the limb, and the circumferential measurements are recorded. The opposite limb is marked and measured in the same way.

Measurements of the affected limb can be repeated periodically in order to observe change, but it is not necessary to repeat measurements of the opposite limb for comparison unless it appears to change for some reason.

Volumetric measurements. Gross changes in the extremities can be estimated by immersing each limb in turn in a bath of water and recording the amount of water displaced. This method is more appropriate to assessment of oedema, but unless there is considerable swelling the amount of displaced water may be too small to be measured accurately.

Range of Movement

Range of movement of joints (ROM) is measured prior to treatment and to assess progress. Measurements may be used to:

(1) record incremental and decremental changes in ROM;
(2) differentiate between limitation of range due to disorder of the joint itself and limitation due to reduced extensibility of muscle tissue or overall loss of length.

Range is measured with movement restricted to the one joint with the rest of the limb in an optimal position in order to (1) eliminate compensatory movements at other joints, and (2) reduce the effects of adaptive shortening of muscles. If range is limited by the length or extensibility of muscles which act over more than one joint, it can be measured as it occurs in a total pattern of movement.

Goniometry. An instrument to measure ROM should be accurate so that it always measures the same thing in the same way; and the method of use should be reliable so that measurements made on different occasions by the same or another assessor are comparable. Sophisticated methods such as polarised light goniometry are available in research centres, and very simple, hand-held goniometers are used clinically. The commonest instrument is the *standard goniometer*, a plastic or metal protractor with movable arms. Its facility opens it to misuse, inaccuracy and unreliability. Skilful use of the standard goniometer and consequent usefulness of recordings require several essential conditions.

Firstly, the pivot and arms must be located as accurately as possible in relation to the axis of movement and the long axis of the moving segments; and care must be taken to ensure that neither the pivot nor the arms move during movement as muscles contract and contours change. When a series of measurements of the same joint is made over a period of time, the pivot and arms of the goniometer should be located in exactly the same place on each occasion so that the series records change truthfully. Similarly, when joints on opposite sides of the body are measured, the positions of the pivot and arms should be replicated as closely as possible so that comparisons are valid. It is difficult to use a goniometer with total accuracy because subcutaneous bony points are rarely defined well enough to provide sufficiently precise points of reference. Performance can be improved by marking the skin with an indelible ink or dye so that the positions of the pivot and arms are repeated as exactly as possible; but all readings are subject to error made by the assessor. Therefore, assessors should remember that an increase or decrease in range of 5° on different occasions or between different assessors is unlikely to be significant therapeutically. The amount of error can be reduced by taking several readings at each assessment, reporting the average, and recording that it is an average of three or more readings.

Large joints can be measured more accurately with the *'Universal' circular goniometer* than with a standard goniometer. It has a biconcave lens which reduces the size of the image, and some models have a built-in spirit level which allows readings to be made with an exactly horizontal level as the base line.

The range of flexion of the hip joint, for example, is difficult to measure accurately with a standard goniometer because (1) the bony contours which might be used as reference points are well covered by soft tissue usually; and (2) it is difficult to isolate movements occurring at the hip joint from accompanying pelvic movement. The 'fixed-line' technique with the Universal goniometer is a more accurate and more reliable method of measurement, partly because the goniometer does not have to be moved as the joint is moved.

Measurement of hip flexion is represented in Figure 6.2. The patient lies supine on a flat, firm, horizontal surface and the assessor marks the skin over the greater trochanter and over the head of the fibula. The patient flexes his hip and knee until the limit of the range is reached. The opposite limb must remain flat on the supporting surface: if it begins to flex, the moving hip joint has reached the limit of its range of flexion and the measurement is taken at this point. The assessor stands some distance away to the side, looks through the lens, and lines up 0° and 180° with the supporting surface (**a**) and the movable line with the marks on the patient's limb (**b**). The angle (**c**) between the movable line and the horizontal surface is recorded.

Measurement of rotation presents problems for which special goniometers have been developed. It is possible to measure rotation at some joints by more indirect means, applying the principles outlined

Figure 6.2: Measurement of Hip Flexion

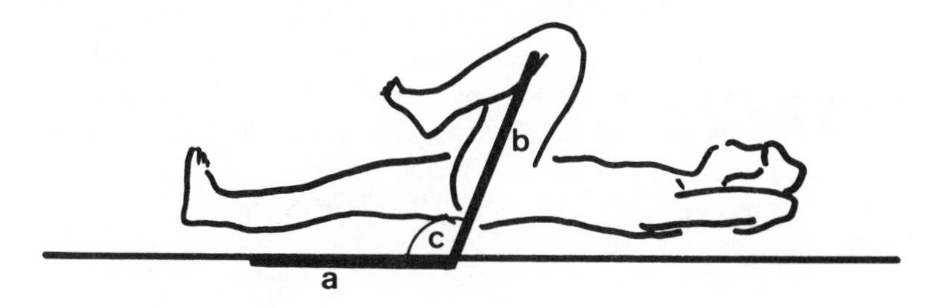

a. supporting surface

b. line from greater trochanter to head of fibula

c. recorded angle

above. For example, rotation at the glenohumeral joint can be measured with the arm abducted to 90° and supported, and the elbow flexed to 90°. With the movable line running from 0° to 180°, the assessor stands some distance away and aligns the pivot of a universal goniometer with the olecranon at the distal end of the long axis of the humerus and lines up the movable line with the long axis of the forearm. The range of inward rotation and of outward rotation are measured from the mid-position. The total range of pronation and supination can be measured in a similar way. The patient sits with his arm by the side, his elbow flexed to 90°, and his forearm supinated and resting on a table. He grips a short stick beyond and in line with the edge of the table and pronates his forearm. In this case, the available range is measured by aligning the pivot with the middle finger, the 0° and 180° marks with the edge of the table, and the movable line with the stick. Pronation and supination can be measured separately by starting in the mid-position.

Recording ranges. For some joints it is appropriate to take the resting or anatomical position of the joint as 0°. For example, abduction at the glenohumeral joint may be recorded from 0° when the arm is at the side of the body; and dorsiflexion and plantarflexion at the talocrural joint can be recorded from 0° when the foot is at right angles to the leg. For goniometry at the knee joint full extension may be taken as 0°. in which case flexion is recorded in the conventional way and limitation of extension is recorded as minus so many degrees. Alternatively, full extension may be taken as 0° for measuring flexion and as 180° for measuring extension so that limitation of extension and genu recurvatum are immediately apparent. To ensure that records are understandable and usable by other practitioners, the conventional method used in a particular physiotherapy department should be adhered to. Whatever method is used, the total range should be recorded for each pair of movements (flexion-extension; abduction-adduction, etc.)

Alternative methods of measurements. Serial measurements of ROM in order to record change can be made other than by goniometry. For example, it is difficult to measure movements of the spine accurately and reliably using the simple instruments in general clinical use. Frequently, a visual estimate is made. While the eye of the experienced clinician has been shown to be an accurate and reliable instrument, estimation is not a valid means of collecting serial readings in order to chart progress. There are several methods by which the range available for functional activity can be assessed.

Using the 'approximation method' shown in Figure 6.3, the distance between two easily identifiable points is measured or an anatomical landmark is identified.

For assessment of side flexion of the trunk, the patient stands with his feet apart and the distance between the mid-point of each heel (**a**) is recorded. He flexes to the side and slides his hand down the lateral aspect of his thigh. Care is taken to ensure that no compensatory movement such as forward flexion or trunk rotation occurs. The distance between the tip of the middle finger and the floor is measured (**b**), or the level it reaches on the limb is recorded (**c**). Measurement is repeated on the other side and any discrepancy between the results can be investigated further.

The distance between two anatomical landmarks or two easily identifiable points can be measured to see how far apart they are rather than how close together. For example, abduction at the metacarpophalangeal joints can be recorded by asking the patient to stretch out his fingers and measuring the distance between the centres of adjacent nail beds. Alternatively, measuring the distance between the medial malleoli will give some indication of the range of hip abduction.

Tracing the shape of a part at the full extent of available range is particularly appropriate to small joints such as interphalangeal joints. Strips

Figure 6.3: Measurement of Side Flexion

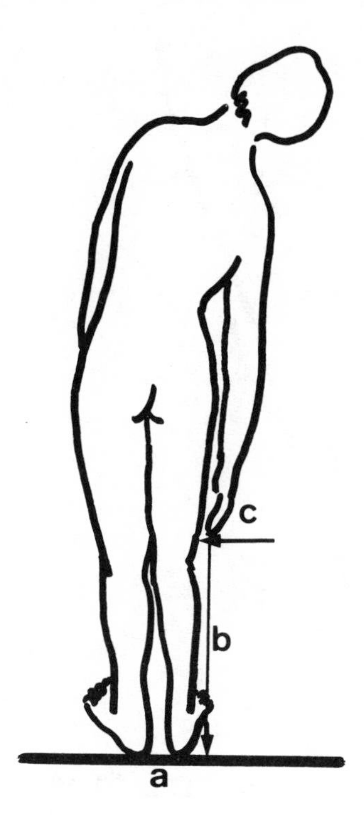

Record

a. distance between heels

and

b. distance between tip of middle finger and floor

or

c. level reached on limb

of lead or multicore solder or a daughtsman's flexible curve are moulded closely to the part, carefully removed, laid on a sheet of paper, and traced. A series of tracings can demonstrate changes in available range very adequately. Assessment of the joints of the great toe is shown in Figure 6.4. The malleable material is placed on the dorsal surface with the end of the strip level with the base of the nail and moulded to the contour of the toe.

Figure 6.4: Tracing of Great Toe

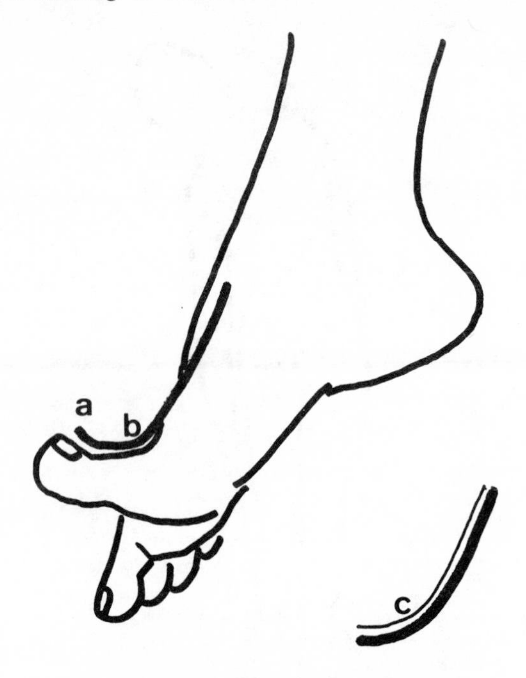

a. place end of strip to nail base

b. mould to contour

c. remove and trace

Malleable materials can also be used to record changes in ROM of larger joints. For example, it is particularly difficult to measure flexion and extension at the radiocarpal joint with either a Universal or a standard goniometer: the two movements have different axes, bony landmarks are indistinct, and carpal movement cannot be eliminated. Records can be obtained by moulding a sheet or strip of malleable material over the dorsal aspect of the flexed or extended wrist as far as the head of the third metacarpal bone.

It is beyond the scope of this book to describe techniques for every ROM at every joint. The methods given can be adapted with clinical experience, and specially developed methods can be found in specialised books.

Interpretation of results. Measurements can be made in order to differentiate between the patient's active range of movement and the available passive range.

(1) If a muscle lacks sufficient strength or if contraction is inhibited by pain, active range will be limited when passive range is full.
(2) If there is some structural obstruction or pain, or fear of pain hinders movement, both active and passive range are likely to be restricted to more or less the same degree.

When ROM is measured it is often assumed that loss or gain of 5° in one part of the range is as important as 5° in any other part of the range. Although this is true geometrically, it is not true functionally. Within the ROM at any joint there are critical ranges which have considerable influence on a patient's functional ability;; and loss of 5° in one part of the range can be more disabling than 15° elsewhere. Figure 6.5 illustrates critical ranges of flexion of the fingers. If the range of flexion at the metacarpophalangeal and interphalangeal joints of the fingers is severely limited:

(1) even if the flexor muscles have enough power to grip, the fingers will not function effectively until sufficient flexion is restored to allow the lines of force to be directed from the finger pads towards the base of the hand and the thenar eminence (Figure 6.5A).
(2) when this range is achieved another critical range is reached when the lines of force can be directed from the tips rather than the pads of the fingers towards the thenar eminence so that the fingers are buttressed together to achieve a power grip (Figure 6.5B).

From the patient's point of view, loss of range is a theoretical consideration. He experiences loss of movement as activities which are impossible, awkward or difficult to perform. He appreciates recovery as he regains the ability to carry out particular tasks in his individual style. Consequently, measurements of range of movement of any joint should be qualified with assessment of the patient's functional ability and posture, and with analysis of gait in appropriate conditions.

Integrity and Stability of Joints

Stability of joints depends upon the integrity of ligaments and the power of muscles acting over them. Integrity is tested by subjecting ligaments

Figure 6.5: Critical Ranges of Functional Movement

A. Holding a ball

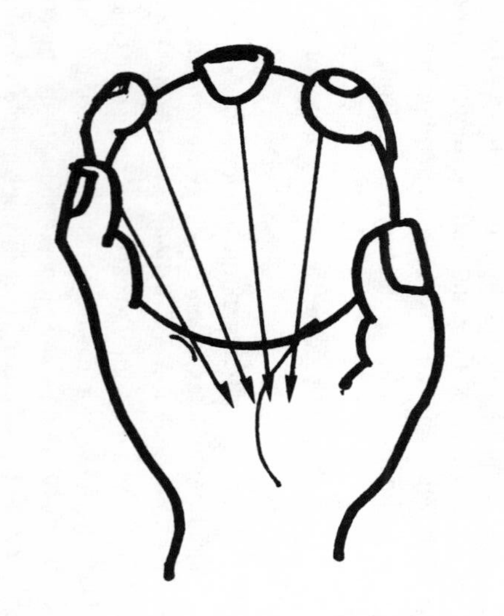

B. Power grip

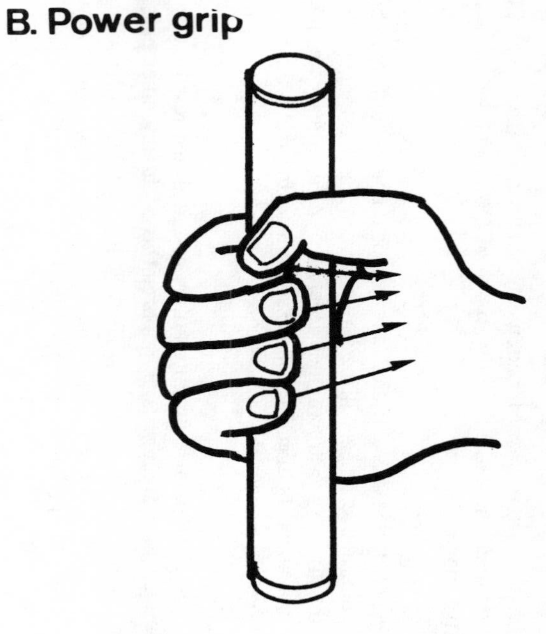

Figure 6.6: Test of Integrity of the Medical Collateral Ligament of the Knee Joint

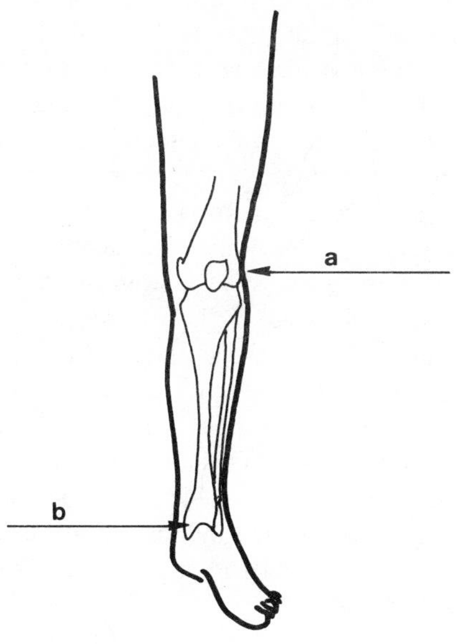

a. **fulcrum**

b. **application of valgus stress**

and other non-contractile periarticular structures to potentially disruptive stress. Rotational, shearing and angular forces are applied to the joint to see whether movement occurs which is normally prevented by specific structures.

Test of the collateral ligaments of the knee joint. The passive test of integrity of the medial collateral ligament is illustrated in Figure 6.6. The patient lies supine with the knee in full extension and the muscles relaxed. The assessor supports the leg by grasping it around the medial malleolus and places her other hand on the lateral aspect of the lateral condyle of the femur. The hand on the femur acts as a fulcrum (**a**) and an abduction force (valgus stress) is applied to the tibia (**b**). There will be no movement unless the integrity of the joint is compromised. If the ligament is torn, the medial aspect of the joint will open: if it is strained, the joint will remain stable but the stress will cause pain. The lateral ligament is tested by applying an adduction force (varus stress) to the lower end of the tibia with one hand over the medial condyle of the femur to act as the fulcrum.

Test of the cruciate ligaments of the knee joint. The anterior and posterior cruciate ligaments are tested with the knee flexed to a right angle, the heel fixed on the plinth, and the muscles relaxed. (The assessor can sit on the patient's foot to make sure that it does not move during the test.) The fingers of both hands are interlocked behind the upper end of the tibia, the thumbs are fixed on the femoral condyles and the upper end of the tibia is moved backwards and forwards. The anterior cruciate ligament is damaged if there is more than a quarter of an inch of forward movement (or more movement than is available on the opposite side if it is sound). If there is excessive movement backwards, the posterior cruciate ligament is affected similarly.

Stability of the lower limb is of such importance during weight-bearing activities that joints of the lower limb should be tested when they are compressed by bearing weight. The greater stress may reveal instability which is not apparent when joints are tested passively. The knee joint, for example, is particularly vulnerable to rotational stresses when the heel is fixed by weight-bearing. The pull of gravity is an important element in the typical waddling Trendelenburg gait caused by postural instability of the pelvis on the femoa.

Trendelenburg test. This is a test of the weight-bearing side. The assessor stands behind the patient and, if the disorder is unilateral, asks the patient to stand on the sound leg and lift the other leg. She inspects the tilt of the pelvis, and then puts one hand on the iliac crest on the non-weight-bearing side and asks the patient to repeat the movement. The test is repeated on the other side. The pelvis should rise on the non-weight-bearing side (Figure 6.7:A) due to the coupled action of the side flexor muscles of the trunk on the non-weight-bearing side and the abductor muscles of the hip on the weight-bearing side. It may fall on the non-weight-bearing side (Figure 6.7:B) for several different reasons. If the abductor muscles are paralysed, by poliomyelitis for example, or profoundly weak, the side flexors alone will be unable to stabilise the pelvis. If the greater trochanter is displaced upwards due to coxa vara or congenital dislocation of the hip, the abductors will be actively insufficient to perform the task because their insertion is approximated to their origin. If the fulcrum of the movement is unstable, due to un-united fracture of the neck of femur, for example, the muscles will be unable to stabilise the pelvis properly and adequately.

Figure 6.7: Trendelenburg Test

A. Normal

pelvis rises

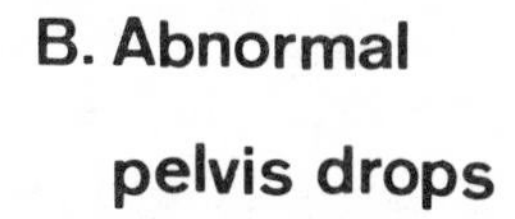

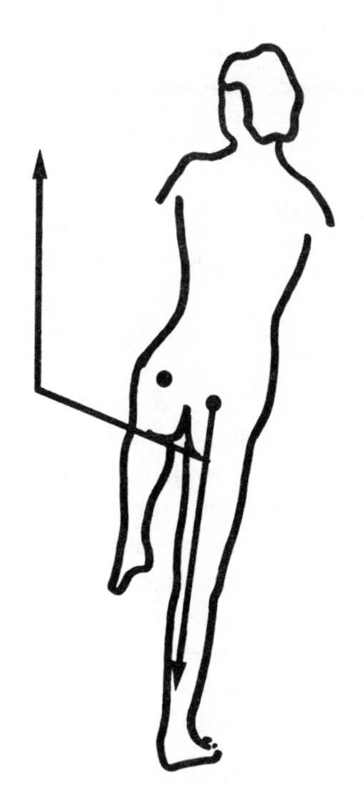

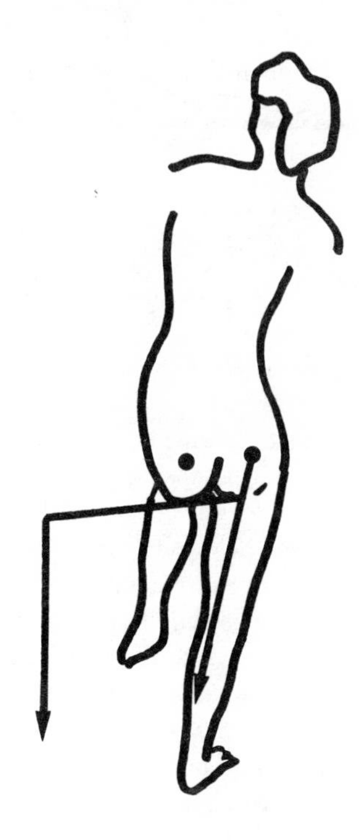

Acquired Joint Deformity

The patient's condition or observation of gait and posture may suggest deformity of one or more joints. Deformities of the hip joint can be examined.

Test for fixed flexion deformity of the hip (Figure 6.8). For Thomas's test, the patient lies supine and the assessor tries to place her hand underneath his lumbar spine. If there is no lordosis and the patients' thighs are in

Figure 6.8: Test for Fixed Flexion Deformity of Hip Joint

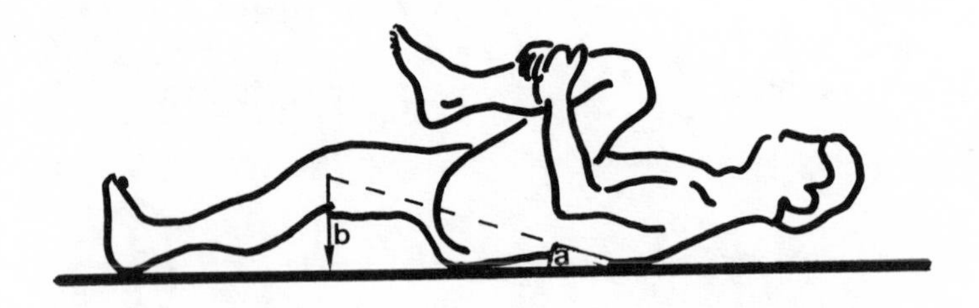

Record

a. angle between thigh and plinth

or

b. perpendicular distance from adductor tubercle

contact with the supporting surface there is no flexion deformity of the hip joint. Conversely, the lumbar spine will be lordotic if the pelvis is rotated forwards in order for the thighs to touch the plinth. The amount of fixed deformity can be estimated if the patient holds the thigh (on the sound side if one hip is affected) against the abdominal wall, or as close to it as possible, to ensure that the hip is fully flexed, the lumbar spine is flattened and the pelvis is stable. Normally, the limb under test will remain flat on the plinth with the hip joint in full extension. Fixed flexion deformity will cause the thigh to lose contact with the plinth. The angle between the thigh and the supporting surface or the perpendicular distance from the adductor tubercle to it can be measured.

Test for fixed lateral rotation deformity. In the resting position of the lower limb in supine the patella is normally directed forwards. Fixed lateral rotation deformity will prevent the assessor rolling the limb to achieve the position of neutral rotation.

Test for fixed adduction deformity of the hip joint. Observe the patient lying supine on a firm surface with the lower limbs more or less parallel. The transverse plane of the pelvis should make an angle of 90° with an imaginary line parellel to the line of gravity (Figure 6.9:A). If there is a fixed adduction deformity of one hip (Figure 6.9:B), the transverse plane $(x - x^1)$ will make an obtuse angle with the imaginary line $(y - y^1)$

Figure 6.9: Test for Fixed Adduction Deformity of Hip Joint

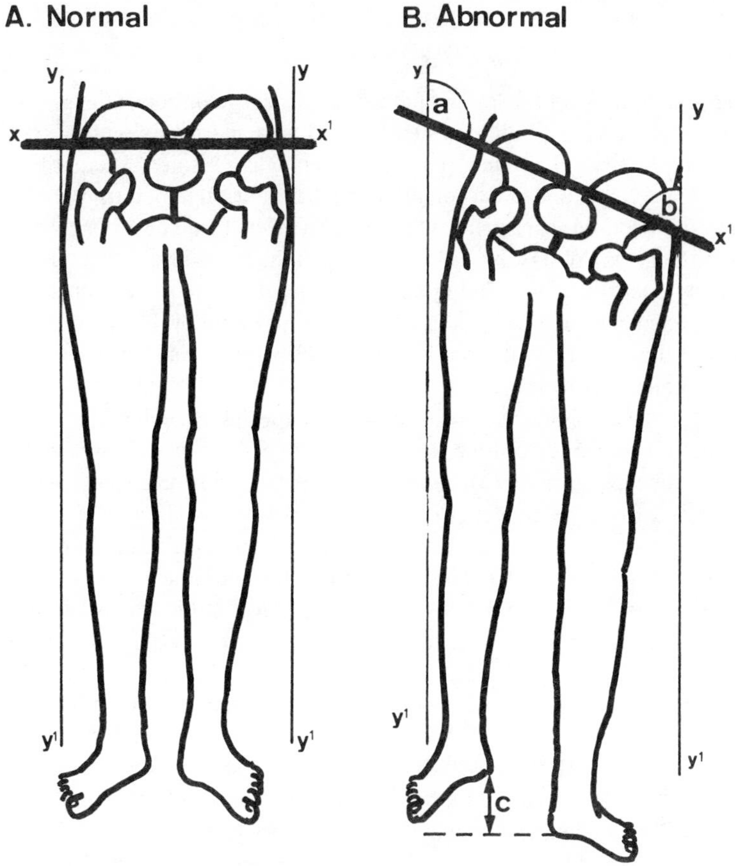
A. Normal
B. Abnormal
y
y
x
x¹
y¹
y¹
y
a
y
b
x¹
y¹
c
y¹

x–x¹ transverse plane of pelvis

y–y¹ line parallel to line of gravity

a obtuse angle on deformed side

b acute angle on sound side

c apparent shortening

on the side of the deformed hip (**a**) and an acute angle on the sound side (**b**) because the pelvis is tilted laterally to the sound side. The affected limb will appear short (**c**).

Measurement of Length of the Lower Limb

True shortening of the lower limb may occur above or below the greater trochanter due to conditions such as coxa vara and malunion of a fracture of the shaft of femur. Apparent shortening is a result of lateral tilting of the pelvis secondary to conditions such as abduction deformity of the hip joint and lumbar scoliosis. Both apparent and true discrepancies in limb length are observable as lateral tilting of the pelvis in standing. Lateral tilting due to true shortening and deformity of the hip is eliminated if the patient sits on a hard seat such as a gymnastic stool. Both the lateral tilt of the pelvis and the scoliosis will still be observable if the patient has lumbar scoliosis.

Three measurements may be made to the medial malleolus (**d**) on each limb in order to determine the level of any discrepancy (Figure 6.10): from the xiphisternum (**a**); from the anterior superior iliac spine (ASIS) (**b**); and from the greater trochanter (**c**). The proximal end of the tape measure should be placed distal to the bony landmark, pushed up to it, and held with the thumb. The distal end of the tape is held in an inferior pincer grip so that the index finger can be placed immediately distal to the medial malleolus and the measurement can be read against the thumb nail.

Measurements are made with the patient supine on a firm surface. The assessor palpates both ASISs to determine whether or not the pelvis is set square with the lower limbs. If it is not, she must try to correct the alignment so that the limbs are in neutral and similarly disposed to the pelvis. If alignment cannot be corrected because one limb cannot be placed in neutral, *the other limb must be abducted or adducted through a corresponding angle before true length is measured.*

True length of limb. This is measured from the ASIS to the medial malleolus, because there is no suitable surface landmark over the centre of the acetabulum. Even if there is an abduction or adduction deformity of one hip, measurements of both limbs will be comparable *as long as the other limb has been abducted or adducted to a corresponding degree.*

Site of true shortening. This can be estimated by measuring from the greater trochanter to the medial malleolus on each side. If a discrepancy

Figure 6.10: Measurement of Limb Length

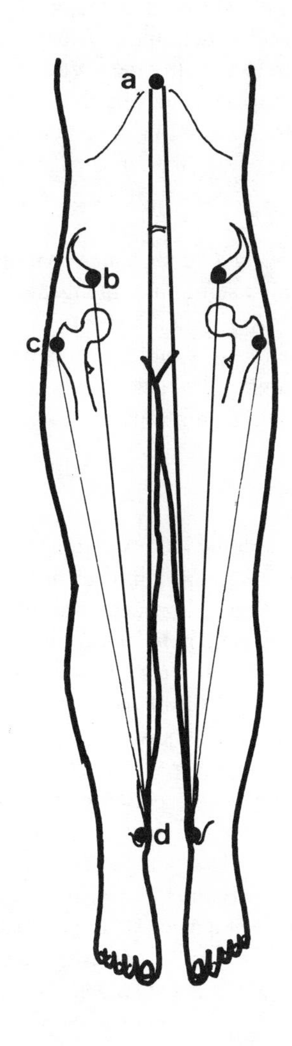

a. xiphisternum   b. anterior superior iliac spine

c. greater trochanter   d. medial malleolus

is found, individual measurements should be made from the greater trochanter to the line of the knee joint and from the line of the knee joint to the medial malleolus on each limb to determine if the femur or the tibia is short. If there is no discrepancy in the measurements, the site of shortening is above the level of the trochanter (e.g. following fracture of the neck of femur). Other tests, such as measurement of Bryant's triangle and construction of Nelaton's line and Schoemaker's lines, can be made to examine true shortening above the trochanter.

Apparent shortening. If the pelvis cannot be set square with the limbs, measurements are made from the xiphisternum to the medial malleolus on each side *with the limbs parallel*. Apparent discrepancy is always due to sideways tilting of the pelvis as a result of either abduction or adduction deformity of the hip joint or lumbar scoliosis. Measurements from the ASIS to the medial malleolus with the limbs parallel will be unequal also.

Special Tests of the Spine

Assessment of the spine includes procedures for examining the cervical, thoracic and lumbosacral regions, the sacroiliac joints and the limb girdles. The majority of the following tests assess the freedom of movement of the spinal roots and their dural sleeves; and none of them will cause pain if the structures are normally extensible. It must be remembered that it is difficult to control spinal rotation and tilt of the pelvis and that the manoeuvres stress joints also. Results can be equivocal, especially if joints are irritable. Consequently, both the conduct of the tests and the interpretation of results require supervision by an experienced physiotherapist.

Straight leg raise and knee extension. These tests assess the free movement of the fourth and fifth lumbar roots and the first and second sacral roots and their sleeves, with the greatest tension on the first sacral root. If a nerve root is trapped or it must cover a longer distance because of a protrusion, stretching will cause pain in the outer range of the passive movement usually. The point at which pain is elicited by passive raising of the limb and passive extension of the knee allows the severity of the lesion to be estimated roughly.

For the straight leg raise test, the patient lies supine on a flat, firm surface. With the knee held in extension, the lower limb is elevated gently. The point at which tension limits further movement is noted and the movement is terminated immediately if any pain is induced (Lasegue's sign). The available range is variable normally: the angle between the long axis of the limb and the supporting surface ranges between 120° and as little as 70°, and a discrepancy of 5–10° between the limbs is not necessarily significant. Consequently, pain which is felt when the leg is nearly vertical may be a 'false-positive Lasegue's sign' due to stretching of the hamstrings.

For the knee extension test, the patient sits on a firm surface, his knee is extended passively, and the point at which tension limits movement is noted. Gravitational compression increases the pressure on invertebral discs. Therefore, restriction of free movement of meninges is increased in sitting, and is even more limited if the patient slumps forwards.

Knee flexion test. This test stretches the femoral nerve and assesses the mobility of the second, third and fourth lumbar roots, with the greatest tension on the third lumbar root. The patient lies prone, his pelvis is stabilised with his hips extended, and his knee is flexed gently. The movement is terminated immediately if any pain is induced.

Neck flexion test. This test is used to determine the extensibility of structures in the vertebral canal as far caudally as the thoracolumbar region. The patient lies supine. The assessor places one hand on his sternum and her other hand under his occiput and the upper part of the cervical spine, and flexes his neck gently. This test can aggravate low back pain or pain referred to the lower limb. The movement is terminated immediately if any pain is induced (Brudzinski's sign).

Movements of the head and neck can aggravate symptoms of basilar artery insufficiency if osteophytes or other outgrowths are impinging on either or both vertebral arteries in the transverse foramina of the cervical vertebrae. If the patient complains of dizziness, it may be necessary to distinguish between avoidable and unavoidable causes.

Neck rotation tests. Firstly, the patient sits on a chair. With his shoulders held still, he turns his head from side to side, and then, with his head still, he turns his shoulders from side to side. Secondly, he lies supine and the assessor turns his head gently to one side and holds it in full rotation for several seconds or until the patient complains of dizziness. Then she repeats the test to the opposite side.

If the symptoms are caused by movement of the head in space, due to labyrinthine dysfunction such as vertigo, the patient will complain of them when he moves his head but not when he moves his shoulders. It is potentially more serious if both rotation of the shoulders and turning the head provoke the symptoms, suggesting arterial occlusion. Not only should cervical rotation be avoided during treatment but it may be wise to refer the patient back to the consultant if there is no previous record of the finding. The passive test in supine is necessary because symptoms of arterial occlusion which are not revealed by the active test can be exacerbated by sustained rotation.

7 OBJECTIVE EXAMINATION OF THE NERVOUS SYSTEM

Each person's everyday movements, from the most mundane to the very skilful, become so automatic that he does not know how they are performed and finds it difficult to describe them in words. Co-ordinated movement is the product of harmonious activity of the components of the central and peripheral nervous sytems. Adequate and effective control of posture, movement and balance requires intact pathways for sensory information, integration and motor output. All purposive movements are initiated and guided through their execution by a constant stream of sensory information which reaches the brain from the wide variety of receptors in the skin, muscles, joints, ears and eyes. Additionally, control of movement and balance is so flexible and so adaptive that the brain can generate original and creative patterns of movement to fulfil most requirements immediately. Disorders of movement and posture result from the activity of components which are intact combined with the defective activity of damaged areas and areas which are deprived of their normal output.

Neurological conditions either block the transmission of smoothly co-ordinated patterns to the muscles or cause the brain to generate aberrant synergies. Research in neurobiology is enhancing and modifying knowledge about functional areas of the central nervous system and recovery from trauma. This has gone some way to explaining some of the effects which can be produced by physiotherapeutic handling, but has not yet influenced interpretation of assessments. In order to provide a continuing guide to treatment and to record progress, assessments of patients with neurological conditions, particularly those affecting the central nervous system, face the physiotherapist with three tasks: (a) to record what the patient can do; (b) to describe how he does it; and (c) to identify why the control of movement and balance is disordered. What the patient does, or assessment of his functional ability, must include the subjective appraisal of the patient himself and his relatives or the ward staff of how he is coping in his living environment. How he does it requires observation of his posture, patterns of movement and gait, and comparison with normal patterns in order to identify which components are missing or abnormal. Why he performs in that way may be answered by the physical tests.

The cardinal signs of a lesion of the corticospinal (or pyramidal) tract are lack of control of movement, increase in muscular tone, hyperresponsive tendon reflexes, and the extensor plantar response (or Babinski's sign). The signs of extrapyramidal lesions are more variable: they include difficulty in initiating and controlling movement and balance, impairment of balance reactions, and the appearance of involuntary movement, but tendon reflexes may be hyporeflexive, hyperreflexive or normally responsive and muscular tone may be increased or decreased. The cardinal signs of interruption of the final common pathway at any point are muscular weakness, wasting and fasciculation, flaccidity and loss of tendon reflexes.

Assessment begins with looking at the patient's posture and then handling to feel whether abnormalities of tone are responsible for particular patterns. In order to explain the postural abnormalities which may be seen, tone will be discussed before posture. While these observations are being made, it is necessary to assess whether or not there are concomitant emotional and behavioural changes which will influence treatment.

INSPECTION

General Observation and Palpation

Behaviour and Orientation

Dementia is inability to carry on normal intellectual and mental functions, such as memory, reasoning and recognition. It differs from psychiatric disorders in that it has an organic cause such as interference with neuronal function or destruction of parts of the brain responsible for these functions. It can be caused by oxygen insufficiency in the brain; metabolic disturbances, such as uraemia; vitamin deficiency; toxins, including chronic overuse of drugs; infections; brain tumours; inflammatory disorders; and subdural haematoma. The patient with a head injury may become demented for potentially treatable causes, especially if he has thoracic injuries also, but the dementia may be the result of direct trauma to the cerebral hemispheres. Patients with vascular or degenerative disorders like recurrent cerebrovascular accidents and Parkinson's disease tend to be demented for untreatable causes, as are elderly people with senile dementia and younger patients with Alzheimer's disease (pre-senile dementia) and Huntingdon's Chorea. Several judgements should be made:

Does the patient know where he is?
Is his behaviour consistent with his chronological age?
Does he have an active interest in his condition and treatment?
Is he uncooperative or excessively over-eager in response to efforts to help him?
Is he able to control his emotions?
Is he euphoric or depressed?
Does he behave aggressively towards relatives? other patients? practitioners and ward staff?

In particular, it is necessary to look for signs that he is not aware of his environment or his relationship to it:

Can he formulate a plan of voluntary activity?
Can he imitate gestures?
Is he able to perform routine functions of daily living automatically, such as dressing and undressing?

He may deny his illness altogether because of the perceptual defect known as anosognosia which, like the other agnosias (see 'Perception and Cognition', p. 119), is caused by lesion of the non-dominant cerebral hemisphere.

Muscle Tone

Tone is the elastic tension of muscles which varies between rest and activity. Regulation of tone is dependent on the spinal reflex arc: afferent fibres from receptors in the muscles enter the spinal cord, efferent fibres return from the anterior horn cells to the muscles, and excitation of the anterior horn cells is controlled by supraspinal centres. During activity, tone should be low enough to permit movement yet high enough to withstand gravity. Abnormalities of tone are caused by dysfunction of peripheral or central pathways or supraspinal centres. They can be detected by handling the limb:

How do the muscles appear?
How do they feel?
How do they react to stretch? (see 'Tests: Tendon Reflexes', pp. 101–2).
Does tone alter according to the patient's position?
Is it distributed in particular patterns?

Normal muscle tone does not resist passive movement but appears to assist it and to adjust to changes in direction readily and smoothly. If there is resistance, the muscles are probably either spastically or rigidly hypertonic. If there is no resistance and the limb feels heavy, the muscles are hypotonic or flaccid.

Spasticity. Spasticity is a 'release phenomenon' caused by the release of the antigravity mechanism of the reticular formation from higher control. Spastic muscles stand out visibly and their tendons may appear like cords; they feel abnormally hard; and they resist being stretched. Usually, tone is dominant in antigravity muscles, so that they offer resistance to a greater degree than their antagonists. It may increase when stretch is applied then suddenly collapse to a hypotonic state, like the sensation experienced when the blade of a clasp-knife is opened. It is likely to be at its lowest when the patient is lying on his side and to increase as he becomes more erect. Effort of any type, increasing postural demands to maintain balance, and anxiety can all increase the level of hypertonus. Spasticity due to lesions of the spinal cord is similar in that motor centres of the spinal cord are released from higher control but stretch tends to evoke generalised movements of total flexion or total extension of the lower limbs.

Lesions of the corticospinal tract may also release the phenomenon of *clonus*. It is most evident in the calf muscles and it may be elicited when the ball of the foot touches the ground while the patient is sitting. Slight stretch of the calf muscles causes the hyperactive receptors of stretch to fire and bring about a contraction to relieve the stretch. As the spindles cease firing the muscle relaxes relatively, the heel drops slightly, the calf muscles are stretched again, and the process continues repeatedly, producing rhythmical, fast, sharp jerks. Clonus is a manifestation of hyperactive stretch reflex which can be induced by testing tendon reflexes; and it can be stopped by sustained dorsiflexion.

The term *spasm* is used in several different ways: for example, the protective reaction which occurs in response to pain, or immediately after fracture of a long bone and disappears when the fracture is reduced and immobilised; the non-specific and benign cramp, or tonic spasm, of the calf muscles and interossei which is relieved by stretching the muscles; and the twitches or jerks of clonic spasmodic torticollis. Spasm may be indicative of pathological processes or organic lesions of the nervous system. Infantile spasms are myoclonic seizures associated with significant organic disturbances as a result of congenital abnormalities or perinatal insults. The infant makes gross flexion movements which are aptly named 'salaam attacks' also. In order to obviate confusion when discussing signs of neurological dysfunction, spasm should be reserved for fluctuations in tone. Although it is used to refer to the type of hyper-reaction to stimuli which follows injury to the spinal cord, it should not be used synonymously with spasticity.

Rigidity. This type of hypertonus is due to loss of control of the basal ganglia over the reticular formation. Resistance to passive movement may be regularly or irregularly variable, aptly described as cogwheel rigidity, or it may be uniform through all parts of the range and have a plastic quality known as lead-pipe rigidity. In hysterical rigidity, resistance increases in proportion to the force applied by the assessor.

Hypotonus. Muscles hang away from the bone loosely; they feel soft and flabby; they lack resistance to stretch; and they are unable to move the body or to sustain posture against gravity, but the limbs flop about inertly when they are handled.

This is the type of tone seen in cerebellar disease which results in the muscle spindle being less responsive to stretch and lack of reinforcement of cortical drive to initiate movement.

Muscles may be transiently hypotonic following acute insult to the brain due to cerebrovascular accident, head injury or surgery causing cerebral shock. The sudden withdrawal of descending impulses from supraspinal centres depresses the excitatory state of the anterior horn cells. As the effect of cerebral shock wears off over hours, days or weeks, the release phenomena associated with hypertonus become evident.

Flaccidity. As with hypotonia, muscles hang away from the bone loosely and they may appear small and atrophic; they feel soft and flabby; they are areflexic or hyporeflexic and there is little or no resistance to passive movement; changes in position do not affect the degree or distribution of tone; and the limbs fall into abnormal positions which are limited only by structures around joints.

This atonia or decreased tone is due to disruption of the final common pathway. It is evident when anterior horn cells are affected by spinal shock following spinal cord injury, infections such as poliomyelitis, syringomyelia or vascular occlusion, when spinal roots are compressed by a protruding intervertebral disc or a displaced vertebra, and when a peripheral nerve is impaired by trauma, deficiency disorders or inflammatory conditions.

The terms 'hypotonia' and 'flaccidity' are not always used in a consistent manner, and there is some dispute about the nature of low tone immediately following a cerebrovascular accident. It is referred to as flaccidity if the shock to the anterior horn cells by the sudden loss of descending impulses is thought to be the primary cause, and as hypotonia if the central lesion is considered paramount.

Posture

It is essential that the posture of the patient with a lesion of the central nervous system is looked at methodically. All patients should be observed in supine, unless it is contraindicated or prevented by another condition, and in sitting and standing wherever possible.

Do the two sides of the body look symmetrical in general?
Are the head, neck and trunk in normal alignment?
Is the shoulder girdle or the pelvic girdle or both rotated along the long axis of the body?
How are they disposed to each other?
Are the postures of the limbs more or less the same on each side?
Is the posture of the limbs due to the alignment of the trunk and limb girdles?
Are the postures typical of the distribution of tone in particular lesions?

Decerebrate rigidity. There is considerable increase in extensor tone in all four limbs. The spine is extended and the head and neck may be retracted in opisthotonus; the upper limbs are extended and internally rotated with the wrist flexed; and the lower limbs are extended, adducted and internally rotated with the feet plantarflexed and inverted. Decerebrate rigidity is caused by lesions of the midbrain releasing the facilitatory reticular formation which generates extensor tone.

Decorticate rigidity. A lesion at a higher level causes an increase in extensor tone in the lower limbs and in flexor tone in the upper limbs. Therefore, the lower limbs are in the same posture as decerebrate rigidity but the upper limbs are flexed and internally rotated.

Following head injury or surgery for a space-occupying lesion, a patient may exhibit decerebrate rigidity on one side and decorticate rigidity on the other (Figure 7.1). Additionally, increase in tone may occur in attacks, apparently spontaneously or in response to particular stimuli, such as fluctuations in temperature, blood pressure, pulse rate or respiratory rate. It may also indicate a rise in intracranial pressure. Although the physiotherapist is principally concerned with respiratory care of deeply

Figure 7.1: Decorticate and Decerebrate Posturing

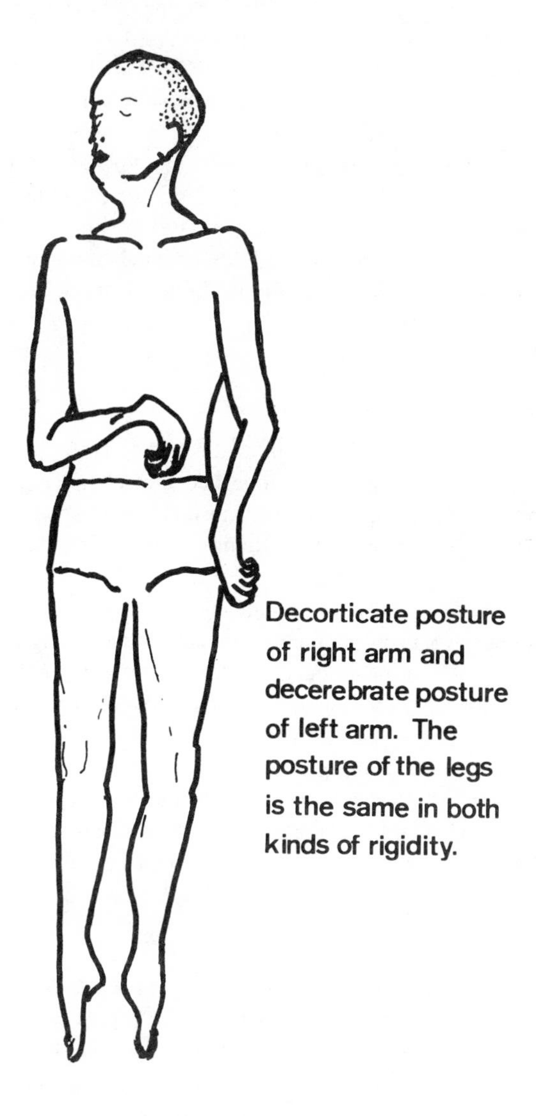

comatose patients who are monitored constantly in intensive care units, she must also be able to recognise the signs of cerebral compression.

Commonly, hemiplegic patients have hemi-decorticate postures, although there is more competition of patterns in the lower limb and it may not be totally extended. Additionally, there will be asymmetry of the trunk, with the shoulder girdle depressed, the pelvic girdle elevated, and both girdles retracted on the affected side.

Parkinsonian rigidity is usually distributed in the general attitude of flexion of the limbs and trunk, known as flexion dystonia, although there may be no resistance to extension.

Hypotonic and flaccid limbs will adopt postures according to the pull of gravity: they may look distorted or, for example, there may be just an excessive amount of outward rotation of the lower limbs. Low tone becomes more evident as the body becomes more erect when there will be marked postural instability of the head, trunk and limb girdles with consequent difficulty in shifting weight, changing position, and making effective use of the arms.

Quality of Movement

Normally, volitional and automatic movement is fluid and purposeful, monitored constantly, and modified and completed smoothly. Abnormalities of control subvert this normal quality, and abnormal synergies will be apparent while the patient performs simple functional activities.

Spastic synergies. Volitional and automatic movement of spastic hemiplegic patients is stereotyped in abnormal synergies which commonly involve the antigravity muscles: depression and retraction of the shoulder girdle, internal rotation and adduction of the arm, flexion of the elbow, wrist and fingers, and pronation of the forearm; and elevation and retraction of the pelvic girdle, extension and internal rotation of the lower limb, and plantarflexion and inversion of the foot. These synergies may not be marked at rest but, for example, the flexor synergy of the upper limb will become obvious if the patient reaches out for an object or while he is walking or performing a difficult task with the other hand (see 'Associated Reactions', p. 104).

Bradykinesia. Independent of their rigidity, Parkinsonian patients initiate and perform movements very slowly. This is associated with loss of automatic movements, such as swinging the arms while walking, and spontaneous movements, such as facial expressions and gestures with the hands. It may progress to akinesia or inability to initiate willed movement at all, which is seen intermittently in patients who suddenly freeze while they are walking. Both bradykinesia and rigidity are caused by depletion of dopamine in the central pathways connecting the basal ganglia which deploy it as a neurotransmitter.

Ataxic dyssynergia. The patterns of movement of ataxic patients are characterised by lack of co-operation between agonists, antagonists, synergists and fixators. The movements are jerky and ill-timed and broken up into their component parts. Sensory ataxia results in delayed and imperfect monitoring of movements in progress. Cerebellar dysfunction causes imperfect correlation of information so that distance and range are imperfectly estimated (dysmetria) and appropriate corrections or modifications are not made as the movement progresses. Additionally, the patient is unable to brake a movement gradually or instantly by contraction of antagonists. For example, the arm may shoot out towards an object, jerk around if the direction needs to be changed, and circle about the target before finally homing in. Mildly ataxic patients may restrict movement voluntarily in order to cope with imperfect postural control. For example, they manipulate objects very close to the chest in order to avoid disturbing the centre of gravity too much. When they are forced to make wider movements of greater range, they try to overcome poor balance reactions by moving very quickly. Ataxia, or its full extent, may not be immediately evident unless the patient is caused to move more slowly, to change direction during the movement, and to stop in different parts of the range.

Involuntary Movement

Involuntary movement may be observed at rest or accompanying movement, usually associated with disorders of the extrapyramidal system. Chorea denotes purposeless sequences of different patterns of movement strung together or embellishing voluntary movement. It is a manifestation of deep-seated lesions of the cerebral hemispheres, Sydenham's Chorea or St Vitus' Dance following rheumatic fever, and Huntingdon's Chorea, a type of inherited pre-senile dementia. Tremor denotes regular or irregular oscillating movements. Fine, rapid tremor is often seen during movement as well as at rest when someone is anxious. Some coarse tremors of the periphery which are relieved somewhat by movement are associated with senility, and others which are relieved by movement but exacerbated by increased postural demands are familial and benign. Hysterical tremor tends to involve the whole limb or whole body and usually worsens if the assessor tries to control it.

Intention tremor describes oscillation of the extremities of cerebellar origin. As the name suggests, it is absent at rest but present during movement. It is marked during fine movements of the fingers and, independent of dysmetria, becomes worse as the reaching hand approaches its target. Nystagmus is an intention tremor of the eyes.

Parkinsonian tremor has two components. A rapidly alternating resting tremor is visible in the tongue and the jaw and as 'pin-rolling' between the index finger and thumb. It disappears during sleep and true relaxation, and anxiety and stress make it more obvious. As it is a resting tremor, it disappears during voluntary movement, but it tends to be replaced by a faster tremor which may progress to the generalised shaking of 'paralysis agitans'.

Gait

The type of analysis described for locomotor assessment is appropriate, and the following points should be noted also:

Can the patient achieve a suitable starting position in sitting from which he can stand up with good postural alignment?
Does he walk in a straight line?
Does he swing his arms reciprocally?
Can he stop and then start walking again?
Can he turn and how does he do it?
Can he negotiate obstacles?
Does he tend to fall, and in what direction?
Is his gait characteristic of a particular condition?

Hemiplegic gait. The principal problem for hemiplegic patients is lack of rotation of the trunk: both the shoulder girdle and the pelvic girdle are retracted and the trunk is flexed towards the hemiplegic side. Consequently, they move the side in one piece, with no rotation between the shoulders and the hips. The affected lower limb is likely to be rigidly extended in order to bear weight, with the weight transmitted through the ball of the foot, and the upper limb does not swing reciprocally but the abnormal flexor synergy may be accentuated. Commonly, hemiplegic patients cannot transfer weight over the rigid pillar so they do not step through with the other limb but take weight on it after a short step, release the affected limb and flex it exaggeratedly at the hip and the knee, then totally extend it again, striking the floor with the ball of the foot transforming the limb into a rigidly extended pillar again (see 'Positive Supporting Reaction', p. 103). Alternatively, they lean to the unaffected side in order to release the affected limb which is swung forward in a semicircular movement.

Parkinsonian gait. Patients with paralysis agitans have difficulty in rising from a chair because their weight is too far back. They tend to lean backwards when they are standing too, which threatens their balance, and many of them compensate by flexing forwards. They take the short, shuffling, rapidly accelerating steps of the text book 'festinating gait', as if their feet are trying to catch up with the centre of gravity, and their arms do not swing reciprocally because they lack trunk rotation. They have difficulty overcoming inertia, apparently because they lack central initiation because they respond to auditory and visual stimuli. For example, they can dance to music and walk upstairs reciprocally, but freeze when they reach the top and the visual stimulus of one step ahead of another is lost. They also have difficulty in changing any movement once it is in progress, seen as difficulty in changing direction and turning round once they are walking; but if they are suddenly stopped with a backward pull when they are walking forwards they start tottering backwards and are unable to stop themselves.

Sensory ataxic gait. When the integrity of the dorsal columns of the spinal cord is impaired, the patient's gait demonstrates diminished proprioceptive sensibility. He stands with a wide base, raises the foot higher than is necessary to clear the ground, wobbles on the standing leg, swings the free leg forward jerkily, and stamps the foot on to the ground again. He may be fairly steady if he watches the ground but his gait will deteriorate in the dark. Even when he can see, visual compensation for diminished proprioception is imperfect, so he tends to stagger and to make exaggerated movements with his upper limbs to maintain his balance.

Cerebellar ataxic gait. Dysfunction of the cerebellum interferes with correlation of proprioceptive, visual and vestibular sensations so that it cannot function to predict such events as when the foot will strike the floor or to control and co-ordinate patterns of voluntary movement and balance reactions. Consequently, these patients swing their legs erratically, the head and trunk sway, the arms may appear to be grabbing at thin air, and they reel from side to side drunkenly.

High stepping gait. Patients with 'foot drop', due to palsy of the common peroneal nerve, or the anterior tibial nerve, lift their feet abnormally high in order to avoid tripping over their own toes.

Functional Ability

The patient's ability to perform his everyday activities of daily living needs to be assessed in his home and working environment as well as in the clinical situation. This assessment may be related to the neurodevelopmental sequence which is observable in infants and babies because it demonstrates two basic biomechanical principles which are fundamental to physiotherapy:

(1) Postural control of the stability of the body becomes more complex as the base becomes smaller and the centre of gravity is raised.
(2) As the balance reactions develop in the maturing infant, the upper limbs become emancipated from their role as props to support the body and to increase the size of the base. This emancipation occurs as ability to react to displacements of the centre of gravity, or of the base, or of both together, becomes more sophisticated (see 'Automatic Postural Adjustment', p. 104).

However, it must be remembered that although the balance reactions of neurologically impaired adults can be improved in the way that children improve theirs, through practice in precarious situations which endanger equilibrium, desophistication of balance reactions occurs naturally as part of the ageing process. Additionally, elderly people in particular are likely to have various other conditions which cause them to avoid positions like prone and four-point kneeling. Patients with central lesions should be observed performing the following activities:

Rolling over in bed.
Moving from lying in bed to sitting on the side of the bed.
Transferring from bed to chair.
Rising from sitting in a chair and sitting down again.
Walking, to the lavatory in particular.

Due regard must be paid to sensory deficits as well as to motor dysfunction. Impairment of cutaneous sensations can endanger patients with peripheral nerve injuries if they are not aware of trauma being inflicted by noxious substances, if the nociceptive flexor withdrawal reflex is not evoked, and if autonomic disturbances and consequent trophic changes allow damage to be inflicted at lower levels of intensity than normal. The hypertonic or hypotonic patient may be unable to move away from potential damage. A mild degree of impairment of proprioception makes balance more precarious; and if balance reactions are elicited they may be too delayed to prevent the patient from falling. Balance will also be affected by impaired control of the trunk and the lower limb, and gait will be inherently unsafe.

Communication

In conversation during the assessment the assessor may become aware of problems with communication which could interfere with a patient's ability to respond to treatment. He could be truly deaf and have a hearing aid which he is not using; he may be unable to use language properly and the likely effect on his ability to respond to treatment must be judged; or he may have difficulty in articulating words.

Dysphasia and aphasia. The patient with a right-sided hemiplegia in particular may be unable to comprehend speech at all, or he may be unable to understand abstract concepts but capable of following simple questions and commands. He may be unable to produce spontaneous speech; or he may use neologisms, or invented or nonsense words, or a descriptive phrase to replace the name of an object which he cannot express. Lesions of the dominant hemisphere may cause receptive or expressive aphasia, or global aphasia encompassing both, and the patient may also be unable to comprehend the written word.

Dysarthria. Spastic dysarthria due to hypertonus of muscles of speech causes a drunken-sounding slurring of syllables which can be heard if the patient is asked to repeat the words 'British Constitution'. Cerebellar disease causes ataxia of these muscles so that the patient emphasises every syllable and his speech loses its normal rhythm. The staccato sound of cerebellar dysarthria will be particularly audible if the patient if asked to repeat the word 'artillery'.

Local Observation and Palpation

The patient with a lesion of the central nervous system usually exhibits generalised signs in the whole body or half of it. The following inspection is particularly pertinent to assessment of the patient with a lesion of the peripheral nervous system. Both sides should be compared in a methodical way in bilateral as well as unilateral lesions.

Is the skin in good condition?
Has it taken on the temperature of the surrounding air?
Is there any tenderness or hypersensitivity to touch?

Is there any change in contour, such as denting and hollowing due to muscle wasting?
Do the muscles feel abnormally soft, or hard and inelastic?
Do any joints appear unstable?
Are there any attitudinal discrepancies, such as 'dropped foot' due to palsy of the common peroneal nerve?
Can these attitudes be reversed passively?
Is an isolated movement aberrant?
Does he use trick movements?

Condition of Skin

A limb may feel cold because of inactivity or because of autonomic disturbances, when it will take on the temperature of the ambient air. Autonomic disturbances are responsible for changes in the condition of the skin also. They may be apparent in stroke patients who have diabetes, and when autonomic fibres travelling within a peripheral nerve have been damaged. In peripheral nerve injuries, the skin may feel dry and scaly because sweating is disturbed and it may atrophy because nutrition is reduced. The skin is vulnerable whenever appreciation of sensation is diminished due to central lesions as well as lesions of the peripheral nerves, and there may be burns or bruises of which the patient is quite unaware.

Pain

Recent research has produced a great deal of information about the nature of the 'pain gate' and inability to close it, particularly after the avulsion of roots (see Melzack and Wall's *The Challenge of Pain*). Particular features of pain tend to be characteristic of particular neurological conditions: irritation of nerves and their roots causes shooting pains which can be induced by traction forces (see 'Locomotor Tests', p. 81); pain caused by a prolapsed disc tends to be aggravated by any activity which increases intraspinal pressure, such as sneezing, straining or coughing; and damage to peripheral nerves causes intractable and persistent 'neuralgic' pain. Neuralgic facial pain can cause devastating symptoms. The face, eyes, mouth, anterior two-thirds of the scalp and anterior intracranial structures are supplied by the three divisions of cranial nerve V, the trigeminal nerve, but pain may be referred to the distribution of cranial nerve I, the olfactory nerve.

Hemiplegic patients frequently complain of pain which is due to traction on the brachial plexus due to poor positioning, damage to supraspinatus or its bursa (commonly due to bad handling), or occlusion of the vascular bundle in the axilla. Severe pain which does not respond to treatment is thought to be a manifestation of malfunction of the thalamus which interprets stimuli as pain originating peripherally. In the 'shoulder-hand syndrome', pain in the shoulder is associated with oedema of the hand.

Muscle Wasting

Wasting is a feature of flaccid paralysis, and therefore of peripheral nerve injuries and spinal injuries. It is not a feature of upper motor neurone lesions, although patients who have been deeply comatose for a long time may become generally wasted and the antagonists of muscles which have been dominantly and unrelievedly spastic for a long time may waste. When atrophied muscles are contracted they look smaller and feel softer and flabbier than normal. They will feel hard and inelastic if they are fibrose, and both contracture of muscles and inflexibility of ligaments and capsules of joints will bring about deformity. Where appropriate, comparative measurements of muscle bulk can be made (see 'Locomoter Tests', p. 66).

Joint Stability

Both central and peripheral neurological conditions can affect the stability of a joint. Ligaments alone are incapable of maintaining the stability of a joint and both flaccidity and hypotonia can result in derangement. Unless alignment is carefully preserved, forces such as body weight, the pull of gravity and the pull of active muscles will stretch ligaments also. Profound instability will be as apparent as the distraction which may be felt between the acromion and the head of humerus of hypotonic patients, or hyperextension of the knee joint or elbow joint during weight-bearing activities. The joint will be vulnerable to damage which causes pain and interferes with treatment of the primary condition. Tests of stability and integrity may be made (see 'Objective Examination of the Locomotor System', p. 73).

Contractures and Deformities

Fixed deformities sometimes result from persistent and unrelieved spasticity causing a limb to be held in a particular pattern constantly. Fixed flexion deformities of the wrist occur in long-standing and untreated hemiplegia patients. Tenotomies of adductor muscles of the hip, hamstrings and tendo achilles are fairly commonly performed on children with spastic cerebral palsy, reflecting the abnormal extensor synergy of the lower limb.

Lesions of peripheral nerves are responsible for specific deformities due to the unopposed action of innervated antagonists of flaccid muscles.

Figure 7.2: Main-en-griffe (caused by injury of ulnar nerve)

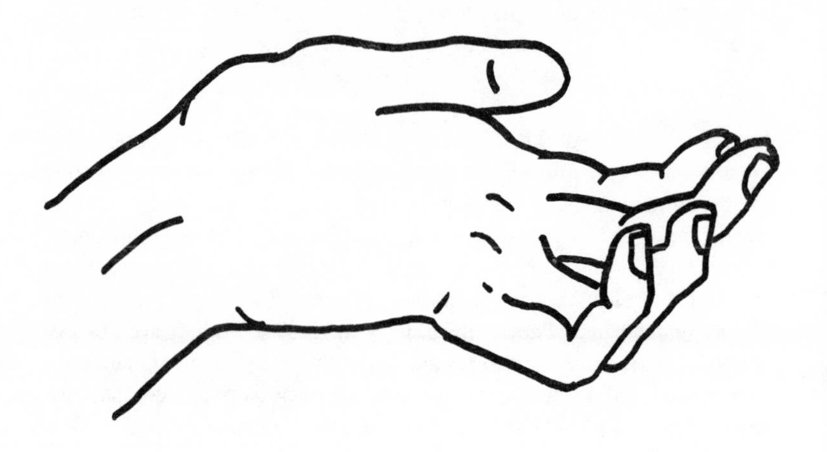

For example, injury to the ulnar nerve at the wrist causes the main-en-griffe or claw hand due to paralysis of the interossei and two or more lumbricals and unopposed action of extensor digitorum producing hyperextension of the metacarpophalangeal joints and the long flexors producing flexion of the interphalangeal joints of the ring and little fingers. This deformity is modified if the ulnar nerve is injured at the elbow and flexor digitorum profundus is paralysed also (Figure 7.2). Anatomical knowledge of the distribution of specific nerves should be applied to analysing the likely paralysis and potential deformity due to the interruption of each peripheral nerve anywhere along its length.

Movement

Loss of motor control over specific groups of muscles due to a peripheral lesion may be characterised by an unusual movement. For example, the patient may roll up his eyeball to compensate for failure of a paralysed eyelid to descend (Bell's phenomenon); or 'wing scapula' may be evident as he pushes forwards with his arms due to palsy of the long thoracic nerve; or he may lean to the opposite side in order to mask inability to abduct the humerus more than 15° due to lesion of the axillary (or circumflex humeral) nerve paralysing deltoid. Most patients will find some way of performing an activity, and assessors must look carefully for trick movements. For example, when the muscles supplied by the radial nerve are paralysed, gravity can be used to extend the wrist in such a way that the assessor can be fooled.

Assessors should bear in mind the observable differences between facial or Bell's palsy due to lesion of cranial nerve VII and facial paresis due to an upper motor neurone lesion. In Bell's palsy, there is paralysis of the whole side of the face, forehead, eye and cheek because the final common pathway has been interrupted, usually by compression within the facial canal. Following a central lesion, the musculature of the forehead is spared and some control over closure of the eye is preserved because these muscles have a bilateral supply from contralateral and ipsilateral upper motor neurones. Sometimes an upper motor neurone lesion affects only emotional movement. Additionally, lower motor neurone lesions lead to atrophy but upper motor neurone lesions do not.

TESTS AND MEASUREMENTS

Motor Responses

Spinal Reflexes

These reflexes are reported in the patient's notes usually, and it is unnecessary for the physiotherapist to retest them if the record is adequate and recent.

The tendon reflexes. These are known also as the myotatic or monosynaptic stretch reflexes, and they are tested to assess the integrity of the spinal reflex arc and the excitability of anterior horn cells. The patient is supported in a comfortable and relaxed position, the appropriate muscle is stretched lightly, and a single, sharp blow is applied to its tendon of insertion. If the tendon is not clearly identifiable visually, the assessor puts her finger or thumb over the tendon and strikes it. The response may be clearly observable as a single jerking movement or it may be felt by palpating the tendon or belly of the muscle. The ligamentum patellae (knee jerk), tendo achilles (ankle jerk), and the tendons of triceps, biceps, supinator and masseter (jaw jerk) are most commonly tested when tone is altered generally. The jaw jerk, which is elicited by tapping a finger placed on the patient's chin when he has his mouth open, is hyperreflexic in upper motor neurone lesions above the level of the nucleus of the Vth cranial nerve. Following lesions of a peripheral nerve, plexus or root, and in progressive disorders, tendon reflexes may be absent or diminished according to the extent of denervation of muscle.

The knee jerk is carried in the femoral nerve via the second, third and fourth lumbar roots.

The ankle jerk is carried in the tibial nerve via the first and second sacral roots.

The triceps jerk is carried in the radial nerve via the sixth and seventh cervical roots.

The biceps jerk is carried in the musculocutaneous nerve via the fifth and sixth cervical roots.

The supinator jerk is carried in the posterior interosseous nerve via the fifth and sixth cervical roots.

Some individuals are able to voluntarily inhibit the knee jerk in particular and others will not relax the quadriceps sufficiently. In either case, Jendrassik's manoeuvre may be required to elicit a reflex even in health. That is, the strong voluntary effort of hooking the fingers together and pulling strongly is used either to increase excitability of anterior horn cells and fusimotor drive or to distract the patient's attention. The responses are graded as follows:

– Diminished or unobtainable (absent) responses are recorded with a minus sign. This occurs most commonly with lesions affecting the spinal reflex arc directly, such as peripheral neuropathy and poliomyelitis. Muscles which are hypotonic (or flaccid) immediately after a cerebral insult do not respond.

\+ Normal (present) responses are recorded with a plus sign.

++ Brisk responses indicate hyperreflexia. This may be caused by nervousness and anxiety, which will be apparent bilaterally. Unilaterally brisk responses are pathologically significant: they are usually associated with spasticity, indicating an upper motor neurone lesion. Hypotonia of cerebellar origin may be manifest as a pendular movement following a brisk response.

+++ Clonus is awarded three plus signs. These rhymthical sustained oscillations may also be evoked by the effects of gravity.

The plantar reflex. With the muscles of the lower limb relaxed, the lateral border of the sole of the foot is stroked from the heel to the little toe. The normal response is flexor: plantarflexion of the lateral four toes, inversion of the forefoot and dorsiflexion at the ankle; recorded ↓ ; and commonly referred to as 'down-going plantars'.

After infancy, the extensor plantar response is abnormal: dorsiflexion of the great toe and fanning of the other toes; recorded ↑ ; and commonly referred to as 'up-going plantars'. This response is known as *Babinski's sign* and it may extend to dorsiflexion at the ankle and flexion of the hip and knee joints. It is always indicative of dysfunction of the corticospinal or pyramidal tract. Therefore, it is normal in babies before they are six or seven months old and the central nervous system is sufficiently mature; it will often be observed in patients who are deeply unconscious; and it will be seen in patients who have had a stroke.

The plantar reflex is part of the nociceptive flexor withdrawal response. Consequently, in progressive lesions, such as multiple sclerosis, the area of excitability may gradually spread upwards towards the knee; and in paraplegia-in-flexion, full withdrawal may be evoked by innocuous stimuli. In paraplegia-in-extension the reflex may be accompanied by plantarflexion of the foot and great toe on the opposite side due to elicitation of the crossed extension reflex.

Positive supporting reaction. Pressure on the ball of the foot to stretch the intrinsic muscles evokes simultaneous cocontraction of flexor and extensor muscles of the lower limb. This is a static modification of the spinal extensor thrust reflex and it indicates loss of higher control over spinal centres. In standing and walking, it turns the leg into a rigid pillar which may bear weight but does not provide the necessary mobility for balance. The negative supporting reaction occurs when the pressure is removed: the limb becomes loose at all joints and free to move again. These two alternating states are inappropriate for activities, such as sitting down, standing up and climbing stairs, in which weight-bearing and movement occur simultaneously.

Tonic Reflexes

These patterns have an inseparable relationshihp with spasticity and it is necessary to attempt to identify them by moving the supine patient's head and cervical spine passively or asking him to perform a movement which will induce them. After each movement, relative changes in muscle tone are estimated, whether or not the limbs have moved. When there is extensive loss of higher control over the centres of the midbrain, brain stem and spinal cord, the patient may exhibit more than one of the reflex postures. The strength of the reaction varies with the level of hypertonus. The response may be immediate when spasticity is strong, although pathological cocontraction may be so severe that antagonists cannot relax reciprocally to permit movement. In a less severely affected patient, there may be a delay of a few seconds before the reaction occurs slowly or increase in tone may not be marked enough to cause visible movement, but resistance may be felt to passive flexion or extension of a limb. Movements of the head and cervical spine may also cause discrete changes in the resting tone of muscles which are consistent with the reflex patterns.

Asymmetrical tonic neck reflex. When the head is turned to one side, there is an increase in extensor tone in the limbs on the side of the jaw and an increase in flexor tone in the limbs on the side of the occiput. Usually, the upper limbs react more than the lower limbs.

Symmetrical tonic neck reflex. When the cervical spine is flexed, there is an increase in extensor tone in the lower limbs and an increase in flexor tone in the upper limbs.

Tonic labyrinthine reflex. Extensor tone is reduced throughout the body when the cervical spine is flexed and increased when the cervical spine is extended. The patient may show marked flexor tone in prone.

Associated reactions. When the patient performs a voluntary activity, such as gathering up a ribbon or piece of paper with his unaffected hand, there is a widespread increase in spasticity throughout the hemiplegic side which may visibly accentuate the hemiplegic attitude or be palpable. These reactions can result from any difficulty, such as problems with speech and fear of falling, as well as voluntary effort.

While experienced physiotherapists can determine the influence of these tonic reflexes by observing the patient as he performs functional activities, it is difficult for the less experienced practitioner to interpret their combined action and to determine which is dominant as the patient's position changes. It requires a great deal of practice to recognise the more commonly occurring combinations. For example, stroke patients may perform various activities with just the unaffected hand and arm and, naturally, they will turn their head to that side to watch what they are doing. The combination of associated reactions and the asymmetrical tonic neck reflex will reinforce the abnormal flexor synergy of the affected arm.

Automatic Postural Adjustment

Fine adjustments are necessary in order to maintain a working relationship between the centre of gravity and the base of support and to ensure that the line of gravity does not fall outside the base to the extent that falling over is inevitable. When this relationship is disturbed by an external force, instantaneous reaction is necessary in order to re-establish it.

Additionally, it will be disturbed by movement, even by movement made to restore balance. Reactions to external forces and the harmonious control of muscular activity depend upon the integrity of sensory organs and pathways, the function of the cerebellum, and the general integration of extrapyramidal function.

The patient should be tested in sitting and standing. Again, he is given a demonstration beforehand. He is moved suddenly with sufficient displacement for the head, trunk and limbs to demonstrate the ability to move automatically and in appropriate ways to restore the centre of gravity to the midline and to protect himself. Assessment of reaction to shifting of weight laterally is particularly important (Figure 7.3). Normal reactions are not stereotyped and, dependent upon the displacement, one of the following types of pattern should be seen. In each case, the movement of the head and the trunk must be observed carefully and the point at which they begin to react automatically should be noted.

(1) The centre of gravity may be maintained over the original base. This is a very complex, sophisticated reaction which demands fine control, and the initial response may be exaggerated and need to be readjusted so that it does not jeopardise balance. For example, if the centre of gravity is displaced to the left in high sitting, all four limbs may move to the right in an attempt to shift the centre of gravity to the right again. If balance is maintained, fine control is used to regain the starting position.
(2) A new, more stable base may be created by an upper or lower limb being extended to increase the size of the base with or without lowering the centre of gravity significantly. For example, when balance is disturbed laterally in sitting, weight may be taken on an outstretched hand with lateral flexion of the head and trunk to the opposite side.
(3) The base may be moved below the centre of gravity as if to catch up with the line of gravity. For example, the patient may hop or step to the side in response to displacement in standing.

Stroke patients may react very tardily, and it may be necessary to wait for a reaction to occur. For example, if the shoulders are moved to the side with the patient sitting upright, it may be several seconds before his head is flexed to the opposite side. Alternatively, it may require a gross displacement before the patient perceives the shift of weight, to the extent that he would be in the process of falling before any reaction occurred. Ataxic patients tend to react in such an exaggerated

Figure 7.3: Automatic Postural Adjustment (to lateral displacement)

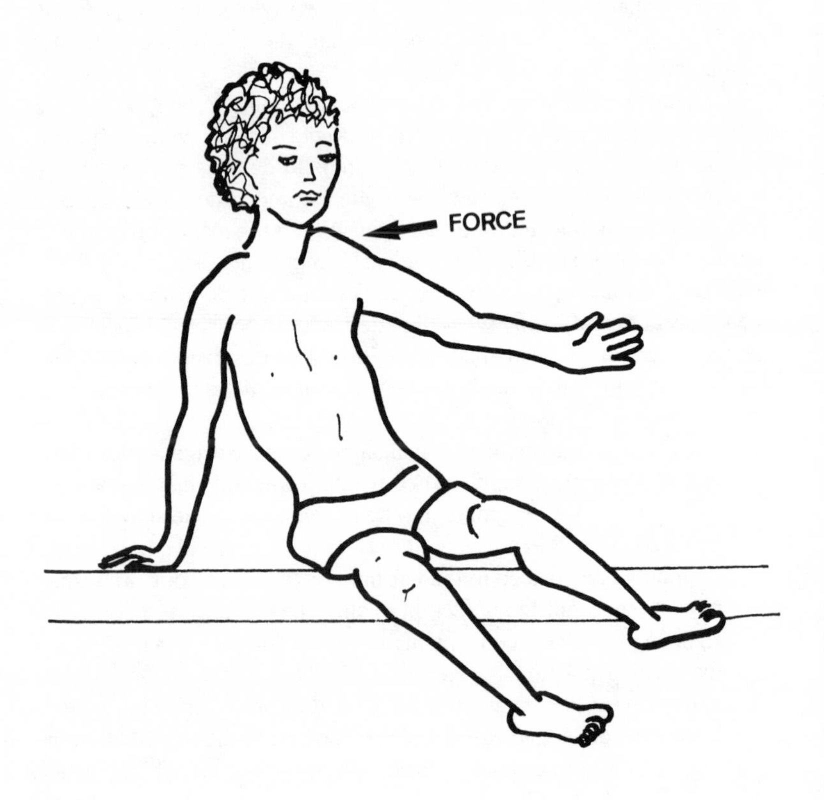

manner that the reactions cause overbalancing in the opposite direction.

Range of Movement

In neurological disorders, active range of movement may appear diminished for such reasons as lack of central initiation of a voluntary movement, inability of flaccid muscles to respond, and hypertonic antagonists resisting a movement. Volitional initiation and spasticity in particular can vary during the day and according to the patient's situation at any particular time, and measurement of range of movement is inappropriate because the range measured during assessment is unlikely to represent the absolute range available.

When contractures are suspected following lesions of the peripheral nervous system, measurement of range of movement may be made using one of the methods described in 'Objective Examination of the Locomotor System' and comparing the active and passive ranges available in the opposite limb. Loss of active range may be due to inability of the prime mover to shorten sufficiently (active insufficiency); and both active and passive range may be limited by mechanical derangement of the joint, contracture of the antagonistic muscle or group of muscles (passive insufficiency), or contracture of other soft tissues.

Muscle Strength

Muscular weakness is the inability to perform motor acts because of loss of normal strength. There are many causes of muscular weakness, including endocrine disorders which affect neural or muscular mechanisms secondarily, primary disease of muscle such as muscular dystrophy causing bilateral weakness and atrophy, and disease of the neuromuscular junction such as myasthenia gravis, causing characteristic fatigue of muscles which are powerful initially.

Loss of control caused by central lesions is often described misleadingly as 'upper motor neurone type of weakness'. This has been responsible for these patients, particularly those who are hypotonic, being approached as though muscular weakness were their major problem. In time, hypotonic muscles and the reflexly inhibited antagonists of spastic muscles may become weak and atrophy with disuse, but essentially patients with central lesions show 'weakness of movement' or lack of cortical drive to initiate and control movement. Consequently, grading of muscles (see 'Oxford grading', pp. 65–6) is inappropriate to patients with upper motor neurone lesions but appropriate particularly to patients with lesions affecting anterior horn cells (e.g. polio), roots (e.g. spinal injury), plexuses (e.g. Erb's palsy), and nerves (e.g. peripheral nerve injuries). It must not be forgotten that a muscle may act as a fixator or a synergist as well as a prime mover or antagonist. As far as possible, each action of each muscle should be observed because a muscle may act in one way but not in others. For example, in hysterical paralysis a muscle which does not function as a prime mover may be seen to act synergistically, as a fixator, or eccentrically.

In different conditions, it is appropriate to record retention of strength and weakness or paralysis according to muscles or to myotomes. Lesions of roots are manifest in loss of strength related to myotomes, and lesions of a plexus also require dysfunction to be identified according to roots.

Peripheral nerve lesions are manifest in loss of muscle strength related to the distribution of the specific nerve and the level of the lesion. Paralysis may be partial or complete depending on the type of lesion, and its duration will vary according to the level of the lesion also. There are three degrees of trauma. The first degree is *neurapraxia*, when pressure obstructs the function of the nerve; the second degree is *axonotmesis*, in which conduction ceases because the axons are disrupted; and the third degree is *neurotmesis*, in which the nerve is severed.

Recovery from neurapraxia begins as soon as pressure of short duration is removed: thus, because there is no structural damage, neurapraxia results in complete paralysis or variable degrees of weakness of short duration. If pressure is prolonged, the axoplasm becomes attenuated and axonotmesis ensues. In axonotmesis and neurotmesis the neurofibrils degenerate proximally to the nearest node of Ranvier and Wallerian degeneration occurs distally. Recovery depends on the integrity of the epineurium and the myelin sheath. Spontaneous regeneration with good prognosis is usual after axonotmesis: thus, axonotmesis of the ulnar nerve at the wrist will result in total paralysis of short duration, but axonotmesis of the brachial plexus will result in complete paralysis of the entire musculature of the upper limb of long duration, and recovery will not be complete unless and until the neurones have regenerated the full length of the peripheral nerves. Neurotmesis results in immediate and total paralysis, and there can be no recovery until the integrity of the epineurium is restored. Prognosis is poor after suturing, particulary in mixed nerves because sensory and motor axons may regenerate anomalously and reach an inappropriate end organ.

In order to determine the level of the lesion of a peripheral nerve or the progress of recovery in root, plexus and nerve lesions, muscles should be tested in the order in which their branches originate from the nerve trunk. As nerves regenerate, pilomotor function is recovered, muscle tone increases before muscles can be activated voluntarily, and muscles function as fixators before they will act as prime movers. They regenerate at a rate of 1 millimetre per day, and the extent of regeneration can be estimated using Tinel's sign. The limb is tapped over the course of the nerve and the patient reports when he feels tingling, which may be within the anaesthetic area. This is usually the level which regenerating fibres have reached and the sensation can be traced distally as regeneration proceeds.

Electrical Reactions

The extent of nervous degeneration and muscular denervation due to damage to peripheral nerves can be estimated using faradic or interrupted direct current. As long as the conducting nerve is functioning normally, all responses to electrical stimuli are brought about by the nerve, and when the nerve has ceased to function a contraction will result from direct stimulation of muscle tissue. However, an intolerable intensity of faradic current is required to produce a contraction of denervated muscle with a pulse lasting for 1 millisecond. Therefore, in practice denervated muscle will not respond to faradic current.

The response to electrical stimulation known as the reaction of degeneration may be partial, complete or absolute. Partial reaction occurs when there is some response to both faradic and interrupted direct current, although a higher intensity than normal is required. It indicates the presence of some conducting fibres and it occurs with neurapraxia, for a short period immediately after axonotmesis, and during regeneration. In neurapraxia there will be electrical conduction below the level of the obstruction but not from above it. Therefore, the nerve trunk may or may not respond to stimulation but the motor end plate will. During the first 14 to 21 days of axonotmesis, the motor end plate will respond to both faradic and interrupted direct current. Once Wallerian degeneration is established, complete reaction of degeneration occurs. There will be no response through the nerve, but the muscle will respond to interrupted direct current. This indicates absence of conducting fibres, and it occurs immediately on neurotmesis. If the muscle fibroses, reaction of degeneration will be absolute and there will be no response at all to electrical stimulation.

A strength-duration curve can be drawn on a graph by plotting the intensity required from either a constant current or a constant voltage stimulator to bring about a minimal contraction applying a series of rectangular pulses of durations ranging from 0.01 to 100 milliseconds (Figure 7.4). The curve reflects the functional capacity of nervous tissue to conduct a stimulus; and, inevitably, a strength-duration curve plotted within three weeks of axonotmesis will provide an inaccurate assessment until the reaction of degeneration is complete. Interpretation focuses on four features:

(1) the form of the curve.
(2) the minimum intensity of stimulus which will produce a contraction if the stimulus is of infinite duration, which is called the *rheobase*. In practice, impulses of 100 milliseconds and above are considered to be of infinite duration.
(3) the minimum duration of pulse which will produce a contraction

Figure 7.4: Chart for Electrical Reactions

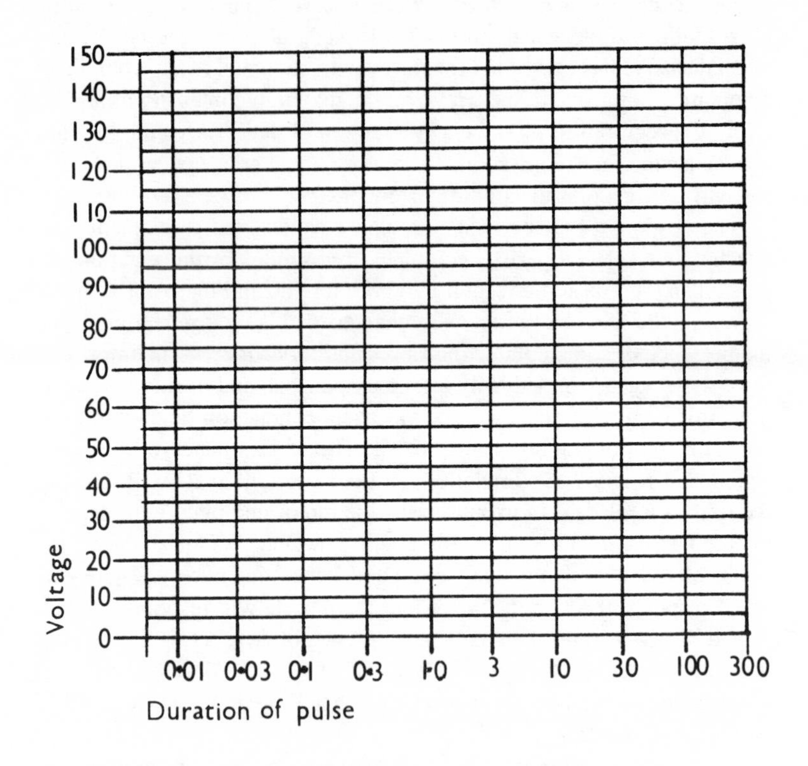

with an intensity twice that of the rheobase, which is called the *chronaxie*.

(4) the relative positions of the curve and the chronaxie to the pulse of 1 millisecond.

Four curves are shown in Figure 7.5. Curve A is produced by normally innervated muscle: the curve is comparatively flat and the chronaxie is less than (or to the left of) 1 millisecond because the nerve responds to the same strength of stimulus whatever the duration of longer pulses. Curve B is produced by completely denervated muscle: there is a steep curve at the right-hand side and the chronaxie is greater than (or to the right of) 1 millisecond because the muscle responds to stimuli of higher

Figure 7.5: Strength-duration Curves

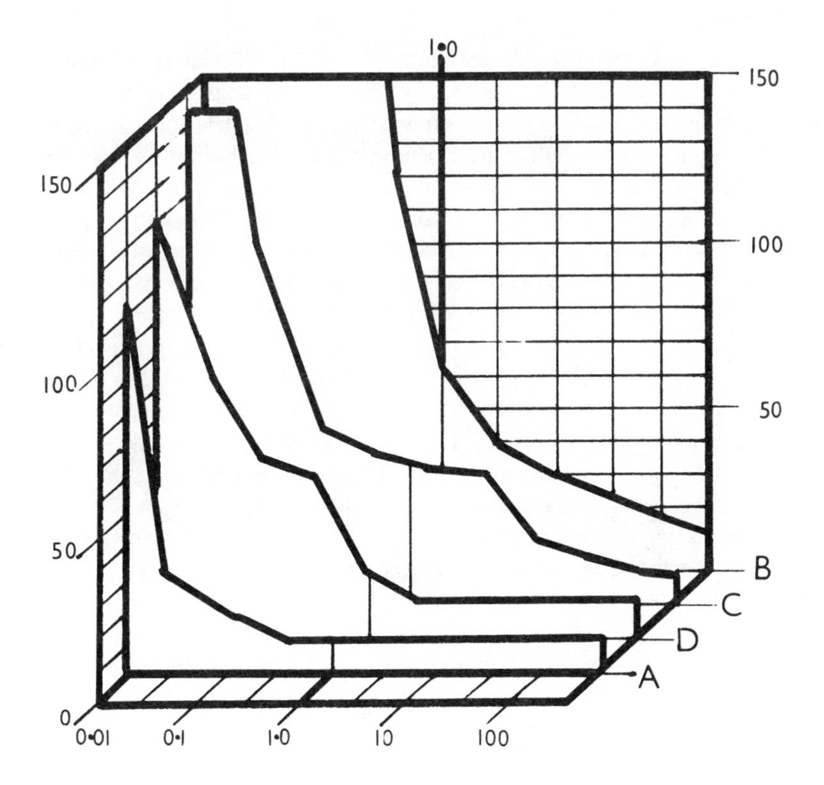

intensity and longer duration but not to impulses of short duration, however high an intensity could be tolerated. Curve C is produced by partially denervated muscle: there are two curves, the curve of partial denervation in response to pulses of longer duration with its chronaxie greater than 1 millisecond, and the innervated curve in response to pulses of shorter duration which is more elevated and further to the left. One test will indicate the proportion of denervated fibres according to the proportion of the curve resembling the curve of denervation, and a series of tests will demonstrate changes in the condition. Curve D shows how the curve descends and extends with the kink merging into the normal curve as regeneration and reinnervation proceed. Conversely, progressive denervation is indicated by an increasing kink moving upwards and to the right.

Sensory Appreciation and Integration

Application of Tests

Altered appreciation of sensation is a common feature of many neurological conditions. Although simple tests will help to define the extent of sensory deficit, it must be stressed that they test the patient's perception of particular stimuli. This depends on the patient's ability to describe exactly what he feels as well as on the integrity of appropriate receptor organs, peripheral and central pathways, and cerebral connections. Patients use a wide range of terms to describe sensory symptoms: numbness, tingling, pins and needles. When listening to the history of a sensory deficit, it is important to identify the type of sensory abnormality the patient is describing. This may be hampered by the perverted sensations or parasthesia which may be experienced, such as crawling and burning of the skin. Obtrusive and uncomfortable tingling or buzzing is a frequent complaint following damage to a peripheral nerve. Appreciation of a specific modality may be diminished (hypoaesthesia) or abolished (anaesthesia) by impairment of a particular tract, and lesions of the thalamus may cause increased irritability (hyperaesthesia). Cutaneous and proprioceptive tests reflect the pathways of the various modalities as shown in Figure 7.6.

Peripheral territories. Lesions of spinal roots result in cutaneous impairment related to dermatomes. Lesions of the peripheral nerves commonly affect all modalities of sensation related to the cutaneous distribution of the particular nerve and the level at which it is interrupted. Partial lesions may show a focus of complete anaesthesia surrounded by a zone of partial loss. The assessor must keep in mind the variation from person to person of the cutaneous distribution of every nerve and the extent of overlap of adjacent territories, for example the anomalous distributions of the ulnar and median nerves in the hand.

Spinal pathways. Appreciation of vibration, movement, joint position sense, displacement of hairs, tactile sensations and the ability to discriminate and localise them are carried in fibres which do not synapse or cross in the spinal cord but travel in the ipsilateral dorsal column before synapsing in the gracile and cuneate nuclei of the medulla. It is important to remember that (a) light touch and pressure, and some joint position sense, are carried in the lateral columns also; (b) perception of vibration through peripheral points is usually diminished with age, in association with desophistication of balance reactions; and (c) care must

Figure 7.6: Pathways of Consciously Appreciated Sensations (from the left side of the body)

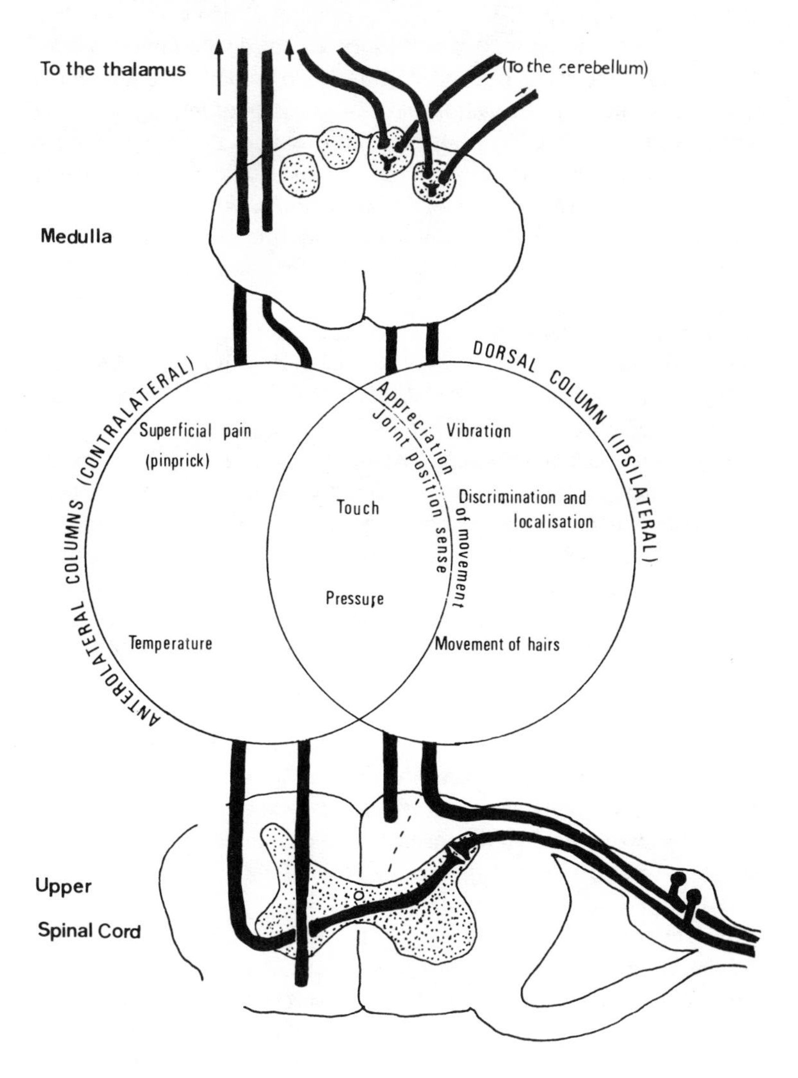

be taken to distinguish between joint position sense and appreciation of movement. Consequently, two-point discrimination is probably the most objective test of integrity of the dorsal column. Patients with multiple sclerosis may show signs both of sensory ataxia, due to impairment of the dorsal column, and of cerebellar ataxia due to lesions in the cerebellum itself interfering with correlation and co-ordination of information. The patient with sensory ataxia is able to compensate to a certain extent for loss of sensory input to the cerebellum with visual information. Usually, he is able to perform the tests of co-ordination with his eyes open but not with them closed and is unable to perform the test for stereognosis successfully, so he will be unable to fasten buttons or to manipulate small objects without looking at what he is doing. The patient with cerebellar ataxia is unable to perform these tests successfully whether his eyes are open or closed. Frequently, signs of cerebellar dysfunction predominate in the upper limbs, neck and trunk, and signs of disease of the dorsal columns predominate in the lower limbs.

Superficial pain and thermal sensations are carried in fibres which synapse and cross in the cord and travel in the lateral spinothalamic tract on the contralateral side before reaching the thalamus through the medial lemniscus. Response to the prick of a pin, to test appreciation of superficial pain, is the basic test. However, tactile stimuli are also carried in the dorsal column and the patient may feel the pressure when he cannot feel the pain. Appreciation of thermal sensation can be tested if the patient's replies are inconsistent.

Light touch and pressure are carried in fibres which synapse and cross in the cord and travel in the anterior spinothalamic tract, and just one of the pair may be tested unless the patient's replies are inconsistent. However, these tactile sensations are also carried in fibres which travel in the dorsal column; and diminished appreciation of light touch might be masked by hairs being displaced.

Central interpretation. The function of the thalamus is to recognise thermal sensations, pin prick and light touch as crude sensations and to relay them to the sensory cortex. Therefore, lesions of the thalamus may interfere with perception of these sensations or cause them to be appreciated as pain. The parietal lobe is concerned with the subtleties of two-point discrimination and localisation of sensation, and lesions are indicated by loss of appreciation of two-point discrimination, sensory inattention and astereognosis, despite successful appreciation of joint position sense and light touch tested individually.

Tests should be demonstrated to the patient and, if possible, applied

Figure 7.7: Body Chart (for recording disturbances of sensory appreciation, pain and tenderness

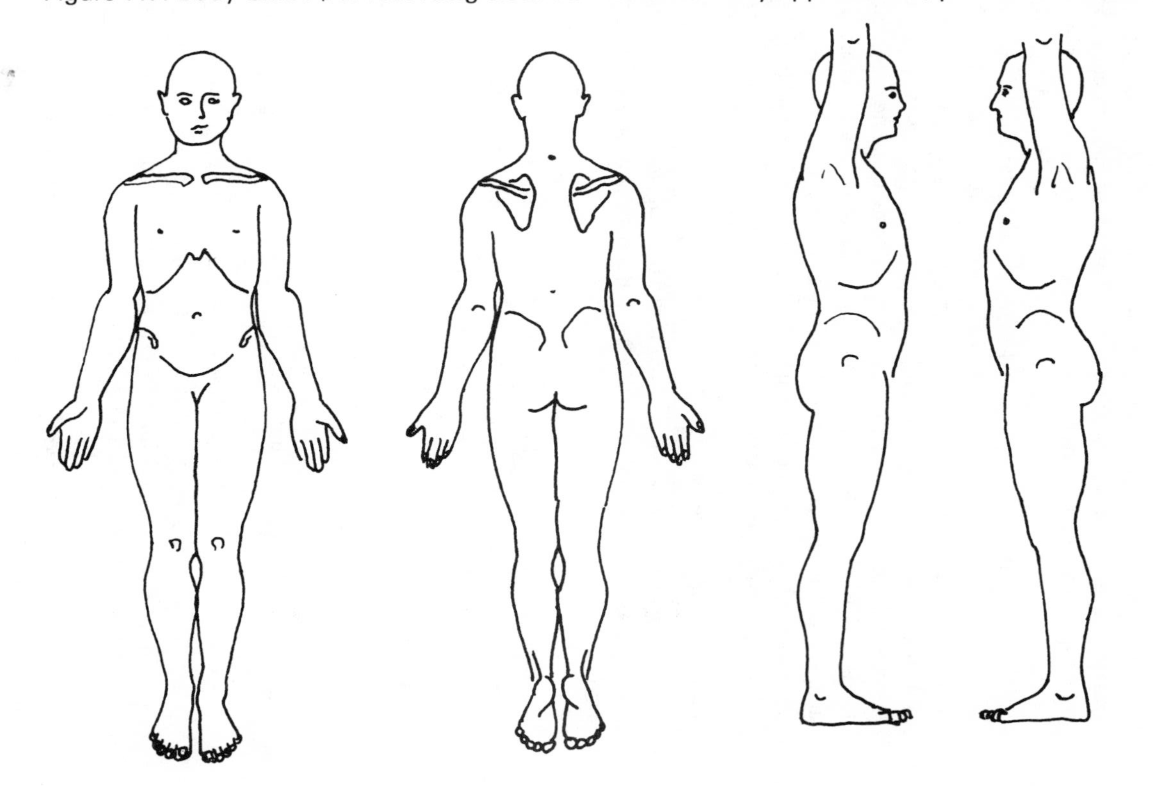

to an area which is normal. Not only is it necessary to ensure that he knows what to expect, but it is inconsiderate to surprise him with the prick of a pin in particular. If he is unable to keep his eyes closed during each test, shield either his eyes or the part being tested. Tests of cutaneous sensation are applied to a normal area first of all, and homologous areas on the opposite side of the body should be tested also. Instructions must be given clearly and concisely and the patient should answer without hesitation. Modifications can be made to accommodate problems with verbal communication. If the patient has a lesion of the central nervous system, the assessor should watch for and note any unusual reactions to tactile sensations, such as complaints of pain due to 'thalamic syndrome'. Partial lesions of peripheral nerves may have a focus of complete cutaneous anaesthesia surrounded by a zone of partial loss. The boundaries of anaesthetic, hypoaesthetic and normally sensitive areas should be defined and recorded on a chart (Figure 7.7).

Cutaneous Sensations

Superficial pain. The skin is pricked with a pin. Light and even pressure must be maintained throughout the test and a normal area is referred to frequently.

Thermal sensations. The skin is touched with the bottom of one test tube containing hot and another containing cold water in random order. If the patient cannot discriminate between them, more receptors can be stimulated by laying the tubes against the skin.

Light touch. The skin is stroked randomly and lightly with a wisp of cotton wool, making note of hairy skin. Following cerebrovascular accident or head injury, patients may demonstrate tactile defensiveness by withdrawing from the stimulus.

Pressure. Even pressure can be applied more reliably with the button of a retractable ball pen. If it is retracted before the patient responds, he is likely to be appreciating pain, such as can be caused by squeezing the tendo achilles, rather than pressure.

Two-point discrimination and localisation. Two blunt points are needed for this test. If dividers are used the points must be reversed, or the patient may respond to the prick of the sharp ends. One point is placed on the skin and the patient is asked to locate it; then both points are applied simultaneously and he is required to determine whether one or two points are in contact. For the remainder of the test one or both points are applied in random order. Normally, the ability to discriminate between two points varies according to the part of the body being touched: usually it is possible to discriminate between points 2 millimetres apart on the fingertips, but impossible to discriminate between points less than an inch apart on the back. Homologous contralateral areas are compared.

Proprioceptive Sensations

Vibration. Commonly, a 'middle C' tuning fork is used. The foot of the fork is placed on a peripheral bony point, such as a malleolus, and moved more proximally if the patient cannot appreciate it.

Movement. The joint is held firmly on either side so that the patient will not be able to feel pressure in the direction of the movement. He is instructed to say 'Now!' (or something similar) immediately he is aware that the part is being moved and to say in which direction the movement has been made. Normally, movement of less than 10° and its direction can be appreciated.

Joint position sense. In bilateral lesions, joints are held in the same way as for testing appreciation of movement and the patient is asked to describe the positions to which they are moved. In unilateral lesions, after a joint on the affected side has been moved to a new position the patient can be asked to describe the position or to repeat it with the sound limb. In either test, the part should not be moved directly to the new position but waggled backwards and forwards in order to ensure that the patient is appreciating the finishing position of the joint rather than the movement towards it.

Integrative Functions

Bilateral simultaneous sensory appreciation. Homologous points on opposite sides of the body are touched or pricked separately then simultaneously, and the patient is asked to identify whether one or both sides are being stimulated. In the case of sensory inattention after a cerebrovascular accident, the patient will appreciate the input from the affected side when it is stimulated separately, but if both sides are stimulated simultaneously he will appreciate only the input from the unaffected side as if it drowns the input from the affected side.

Stereognosis. Place a variety of familiar objects and textures on a tray out of sight of the patient. Place them in his hand one at a time and ask him to name the object or describe the texture. This tests ability to recognise objects by their shape, size, form and texture. Cutaneous and proprioceptive sensations should be assessed beforehand because astereognosis could indicate central integrative dysfunction or inadequate appreciation of light touch and joint position sense. Additionally, stereognosis depends on ability to manipulate an object and closing the patient's hand around it for him will not provide enough information, although he may guess basic shapes, such as a table tennis ball.

Co-ordination

Rhombergism. The patient stands up, reaches forwards with his arms, and closes his eyes. He may sway with his eyes open and closed or only when he closes his eyes.

Finger-nose test. The patient abducts one upper limb then touches the tip of his nose with the tip of his index finger. Alternatively, he can be asked to touch the tip of the assessor's index finger. Whichever test is used, it is repeated with the other limb and with the eyes open as well as closed. Movements should be performed without wavering or random errors. Dysmetria may be apparent as homing in on the target with the eyes open and closed or just with them closed.

Heel-shin test. In half-lying, the patient lifts one leg into the air and places the heel on his opposite knee, slides it down the shin, and replaces the limb on the plinth. He repeats the movement with the other limb and with his eyes open as well as closed. The movement should be performed smoothly and without irregular side to side errors.

A patient with sensory ataxia is likely to perform all of these tests more successfully with his eyes open than with them closed; but a patient with cerebellar ataxia will be equally unsuccessful. Other tests of cerebellar and extrapyramidal function will be found in neurological text books, such as the rebound phenomenon and slapping the hands against the thighs with rapidly alternating pronation and supination to demonstrate dysdiadokokinesis.

Visual Field Defects

Visual field defects may be suspected when patients are surprised by people suddenly appearing in view, or fail to see objects which ought to be clearly in view, or turn the pages of a newspaper without reading the text. Following cerebrovascular accident this is likely to be due to homonymous hemianopia, or loss of the same half of the visual field of both eyes. The patient may be completely unaware of the loss, although patients with left hemianopia sometimes think that they have lost the ability to read also. Text does not make sense because they start to read each line in the middle of the column. This can be demonstrated by drawing a coloured line down the left-hand side of the column so that they turn their heads far enough to the left to start a new line when they can see the coloured line. Both right and left hemianopia can be assessed by testing each eye in turn, sitting half a metre in front of the patient, moving your fingers to the perimeter of your own visual field, and asking the patient to indicate when and where he loses sight of them.

Perception and Cognition

A large class of perceptual and cognitive disorders, called the 'agnosias', is associated with left-sided hemiplegia. This is usually due to an insult to the non-dominant cerebral hemisphere, and corresponding syndromes associated with right-sided hemiplegia are less frequently seen in left-handed patients. The patient may completely ignore activities in the left half of the visual field, or be unaware of the hemiplegic side or part of it and reject it (asomatognosia), or deny the hemiplegia completely (anosognosia). Although they are able to see an object, many patients cannot assess its position, size and movement relative to themselves. Consequently, they are unable to perform simple tasks such as placing the arm in a sleeve to dress themselves.

These problems may be suspected during treatment, and the physiotherapist can make use of the occupational therapist's assessment or devise simple tests to confirm her suspicions. Widespread cognitive and perceptual disorders will restrict functional activities severely and prevent patients taking care of themselves. Perceptual dysfunction due to sensory deprivation and disordered integrative functions can cause considerable problems during rehabilitation of the patient with a head injury also.

MEDICAL DATA OF SIGNIFICANCE TO PHYSIOTHERAPISTS

Many investigations are invasive and there is an element of risk and discomfort for the patient which is increased when a potentially toxic contrast medium is introduced too. Angiograms and air encephalograms in particular are being superseded by the less risky and more informative CAT-scan. Apart from electroencephalography and electromyography, most medical tests assess the anatomy of the brain and spinal cord and their surroundings. Although the information is important diagnostically, it may be only of interest to the physiotherapist without contributing to her assessment or planning of treatment.

Electromyography and Nerve Conduction Studies

An electromyogram is obtained by inserting needle electrodes into the belly of a muscle and recording the electrical activity in the muscle during voluntary contraction and at rest. Action potentials are amplified to provide an auditory signal or visual display to assist differentiation between abnormal muscle and normal muscle, primary disorders of muscle and neurogenic disorders affecting muscle secondarily, and myopathies of varied types.

The speed of conduction of afferent and efferent impulses is estimated by calculating the rate of transmission between active and receptor electrodes applied over a nerve. When a nerve is impaired, conduction tends to be slowed; and when anterior horn cells or a root are impaired, conduction along the nerve may not be slowed until late in the course of the condition. Consequently, nerve conduction tests are used to diagnose compressive lesions of a peripheral nerve, such as carpal tunnel syndrome, and to differentiate between lesions at various levels in the peripheral pathway.

Lumbar Puncture and Myelogram

The subarachnoid space is punctured through either the third or fourth lumbar interspace in order to obtain a sample of cerebrospinal fluid. Normal fluid is clear and colourless and samples are examined for colour, amount of sugar and protein, number of white blood cells and infective organisms. A manometer can be attached to measure the pressure of fluid which is normally 60–150 mm Hg. Pressure will be reduced if circulation of cerebrospinal fluid is obstructed, and occasionally the tap is dry due to complete blockage.

Myelography is performed following lumbar puncture. A radiolucent or radio-opaque contrast medium is injected into the subarachnoid space and the examination table is tilted so that the flow of contrast medium up and down the spinal canal can be watched on a video display. Reports of radiographs of areas of obstruction may confirm evidence of neurological impairment collected during the assessment.

Computer-assisted Axial Tomography (CAT-scan or EMI-scan)

Initially, the technique was called the EMI-scan after the European Musical Instrument Company which pioneered its development, but it is more frequently referred to as the CAT-scan nowadays. The machine rotates in time more than 180° about the head, X-raying the brain from various angles in small slices. The radiographic evidence is computerised and the small variations in projections are compared. The tomographic sections are displayed at very high resolution, allowing visualisation of the shape and density of the substance of the brain. Diagnosis of tumours, aneurysms and other arteriovenous malformations, subdural and epidural haematomas and ventricular abnormalities has improved dramatically since it was introduced.

8 RECORDING ASSESSMENT AND TREATMENT

On the whole, collection of data and recording of information have not been the forte of physiotherapists. In many physiotherapy departments, patients' record cards contain inadequate, irrelevant, or even meaningless data, and some bear only dates of attendances and physiotherapists' initials. This lack of efficient record-keeping is an historic remnant: a persistent reminder of the days when physiotherapists were the handmaidens of doctors, acting as technicians by carrying out medical prescriptions such as 'infrared and exercise three times a week for four weeks' and terminating treatment when the required number of sessions had been recorded.

Physiotherapists acquired two rights when the redefined relationship between medical practitioners and physiotherapists was published in the circular HC(77)33 in 1977: the right to prescribe their own treatment and the right to refuse to carry out treatment prescribed by a medical practitioner. These rights, like all rights, carry obligations: in order to prescribe their own treatment, physiotherapists are obliged to assess each patient adequately and to select treatment which is appropriate and safe; and in order to exercise the right not to apply a treatment prescribed by a doctor, they are obliged to justify their opinion of its potential ineffectiveness, inappropriateness or danger to the patient. Both obligations imply responsibility for evaluation of the effectiveness of physiotherapeutic techniques in the context of total patient care and for efficient use of scarce resources. In order to take advantage of the rights and to fulfil the obligations, efficient record-keeping must be accepted as an additional essential skill in the repertoire of the competent physiotherapist.

Uses of Records

The wide variety of methods of recording information collected during assessments reflects the expectations of different physiotherapists. Just as muscle tone must be high enough to withstand gravity yet low enough to permit movement, so a record system needs to be rigid enough to contain all information needed for current and identifiable future uses and to allow it to be retrieved with ease yet flexible enough to meet individual needs of both patient and physiotherapist. Fowler (1926), Partridge (1957) and Gowers (1977) have given prescriptions for writing well; but, except

Table 8.1: Uses of Physiotherapy Records

1. Detailed aide memoire of personal details, medical history, physical examination,
   laboratory tests and treatment.
2. Justification of selected treatment.
3. Comparison of first assessment and reassessments.
4. Communication to ensure continuity of care.
5. Evaluation of use of modalities of treatment.
6. Clinical research.
7. Pre- and post-registration education.
8. Audits of patient care.
9. Litigation.

for specific instructions for creating Problem Oriented Medical Records, there is very little information of practical significance about the design of records. On the basis of problems consumers have with instructions accompanying various products and domestic appliances, Wright (1981) specified ingredients for adequate instructions: they should be accurate, understandable and clearly structured. She added that the major problem is knowing how to meet the specifications!

Adequate content, presentation and structure are fundamental to the good record also — and here the spcifications can be begun to be met by listing the possible uses of the records. The list of uses of physiotherapy records shown in Table 8.1 is adapted from McIntyre and Petrie (1979).

The Aide Memoire

Concise notes are recorded about the patient's personal details, his medical history and previous treatment, and results of the objective examination and laboratory tests. The physiotherapy diagnosis or interpretation and both the patient's and the physiotherapist's short- and long-term goals are recorded also.

Justification of Selected Treatment

In order to translate the stated goals into clearly defined objectives for any intervention, the individual's medical history and associated treatments, such as drugs or metal implants, must be considered carefully in the light of knowledge of potential dangers of specific treatment modalities. In order to substantiate the choice of physiotherapeutic techniques, the objectives should be recorded as aims and means of treatment or as principles of treatment which reflect knowledge of contraindication and awareness of potential dangers.

Comparisons of Initial Assessment and Reassessments

Patients may be reassessed periodically, such as weekly or monthly, or continuously throughout sessions of treatment and from one session to the next. Periodic reassessment in particular requires a permanent record of assessments so that progress, or regression in some cases, can be judged accurately. Both permanent records of assessments and the continuous record of the patient's response to treatment are necessary in order to justify modification of the programme of treatment.

Communication and Continuity of Care

Well maintained and accurate records are essential for efficient continuity of care when more than one physiotherapist is involved in the care of an individual or when a patient is referred to another department or hospital. They will also contribute to total care of a patient if extracted information is used in written reports to consultants, or if a multidisciplinary approach is utilised and, for example, verbal reports are made at case conferences.

Evaluation of the Use of Modalities of Treatment

Although junior staff are not directly involved in the management and planning of physiotherapy services, their permanent records of assessments and continuous records of treatment which justify selections of modalities of treatment and modifications of the programme of treatment can be of invaluable assistance to more senior staff. Constraints on resources are increasing annually and it is essential for managerial physiotherapists to apply stringent rules to arrange areas of expenditure in order of priority and to justify requests to hospital administrators. Information can be extracted from good records to support claims for investment in additional equipment, specific expertise, or retraining and redeployment of staff.

Clinical Research

The accumulated experience of day-to-day clinical practice is a valuable resource and it can be utilised as a data bank for clinical research if it has been recorded efficiently. Over the years there have been many changes in the popularity of different modes of treatment. Many of these changes may not have been justified. Historically, evaluation of the usefulness of a particular modality has been based on the intuition of the physiotherapist and continued use depended on prescription by doctors. For example, long-wave diathermy is unknown to most physiotherapists under fifty years of age because doctors stopped prescribing it and machines were scrapped before it was ever evaluated scientifically and clinically. Partridge's (1980) statement is patently true: further development of physiotherapy is clearly linked to evaluation of physiotherapy by physiotherapists. Where comprehensive clinical records are kept, information can be retrieved with relative ease and used as a basis for clinical research into methods of treatment. It may highlight a need for changes in approach to treatment; for example, it may be shown that health education is more cost-effective than re-education in some instances.

Pre- and Post-registration Education

Note-taking and record-keeping by students are a source of learning in themselves if used in discussion with more experienced physiotherapists. Constructive criticism can supply important feedback to the student about her clinical performance. Although care studies or case reports are not a feature of *Physiotherapy* journal, they are common in both the medical and the nursing press as a means of general education, they have become an integral part of the education of physiotherapy students, and they are being used much more extensively in post-registration education. Critical appraisal of experiences reinforces the learning process. Care studies teach not only the total management of a patient, his condition and his dysfunction, but also the importance of gathering and recording information accurately. Where accurate records of patients receiving physiotherapy are kept, there is a wealth of useful educational material which can be tapped for all levels of learning.

Audit of Patient Care

Bromley (1978) has written about the 'patient care audit' as a tool for evaluation of the quality of performance in the wider aspects of patient care or to provide a physiotherapist with feedback about the effectiveness of her own performance. It is an objective, structured and sequential analysis of treatment or any specific aspect of patient care. Current practice can be assessed retrospectively or concurrently, but a retrospective audit is feasible only where good records have been kept. When appropriate criteria for the audit have been set and ratified, relevant data are retrieved from the records and subjected to analysis in order to identify differences between expected and actual performances in areas which need to be improved, to plan remedial action, and to improve standards ultimately.

Litigation

Patient records can be an essential safeguard in cases of legal action, when it is necessary to present evidence to the police, solicitors or insurance companies. In civil cases where a patient claims negligence resulting in damage, it may be a case of the physiotherapist's word against that of another or a test of memory if clear, accurate and substantiating records have not been maintained.

Types of Records

Bearing in mind these potential uses of physiotherapy records and applying the principles set out in Table 8.2, it should not be difficult to produce a protocol which would be generally acceptable to those who would be expected to use it. A fairly standard format facilitates ease of use by familiarity, but it should allow flexibility so that it can be modified to meet needs of the individual. The essence of a good record is that material is presented simply and effectively. Just like the face to face interaction between the patient and the practitioner, one of the principal functions of the record is communication. In this case, information is conveyed in a written form which Waller (1979) described as having three functions:

(1) the *enabling function* which provides a clear channel of information;
(2) the *aesthetic function* which provides an attractive reading environment;
(3) the *access function* which identifies and structures particular aspects of the text.

Basically, it is a question of how users with different aims can be enabled to gain access to the information they want. There is no simple answer to this question, because in some situations the record may never be read by anyone other than the physiotherapist who compiles it, in some it may be shown to the patient and discussed with him, and in some it may be referred to by practitioners of other professions.

Loftus, Freedman and Loftus (1970) showed that people find it easier to read and remember familiar words. One difficulty with such words is that they may not have universally consistent meaning. Although it may be assumed that health care practitioners share a common 'medical language', each profession uses language in a way which may appear idiosyncratic or confusing to members of another profession. 'Weakness'

Table 8.2: Principles of Retrieving Information from Physiotherapy Records

1. Record must be readily available.
2. Its information must be:
   (a) understandable
   (b) correct and 'in-context'
   (c) adequate
3. For ease of location and assimilation of information, it should:
   (a) follow a broadly standard format
   (b) demonstrate *key* points
   (c) record *relevant* material only
   (d) be concise
   (e) retain meaning

is a very obvious example which has been discussed in the 'Objective Examination of the Nervous System'. The language of physiotherapy includes such terms as 'diagonal patterns' and 'quality of movement' which are used in conventional senses known only to those whom Gowers (1977) called 'parties to the convention'. The terms are unambiguous shorthand for physiotherapists, but they may be unintelligible to outsiders to whom they have not been explained. Therefore, if a record is required to convey information to members of other professions, such terms must be explained so that they are readily understandable by them.

Critchley (1953) wrote that 'no simple system of marking can possibly replace the full and faithful recording in a descriptive fashion of exactly what the patient says and does under performance. Qualitative changes in behaviour can only in this way be given their true value'. Whatever skills health care practitioners possess, the skill of writing clearly and concisely is rarely one of them. Consequently, narrative accounts are not necessarily more truthful descriptions of patients' dysfunctions than less discursive notes, and they tend to be skipped through because of the time required to read them thoroughly. There are three main types of records in current use, and each is preferred or rejected by physiotherapists working in different situations.

Source-orientated Accounts

An example of a source-orientated record is shown in Figure 8.1. It was drawn up for students to use during their first clinical placements and, consequently, it reflects the structure of the 'Guides to Assessment'. To facilitate learning, a basic pattern is required which imposes uniformity but avoids omissions. It must also be capable of catering to people with different levels of skill and experience. Students must be enabled to apply their increasing experience and skills and, therefore, more senior

Figure 8.1: Source-orientated Record Form

SHEFFIELD CITY POLYTECHNIC
Department of Health Studies

PHYSIOTHERAPY ASSESSMENT

HOSPITAL | WARD/OPD | PATIENT'S NAME | HOSPITAL NUMBER

GP | CONSULTANT | ADDRESS

DATE OF NEXT CONSULTANT/
GP APPOINTMENT

STUDENT PHYSIOTHERAPIST | DATE OF BIRTH | AGE | SEX | CIVIL STATE

DATE OF FIRST ASSESSMENT	MEDICAL DIAGNOSIS

HISTORY
OF PRESENT COMPLAINT

SOCIAL

OF PREVIOUS MEDICAL CONDITION

OBSERVATION
GENERAL

LOCAL

(Figure 8.1 contd.)

DATE	PALPATION
	MOVEMENTS
	TESTS AND INVESTIGATIONS
	FUNCTIONAL ASSESSMENT
	INTERPRETATION (from Assessment)

Figure 8.1 (contd.)

<table>
<tr><td colspan="2" rowspan="2">SHEFFIELD CITY POLYTECHNIC
Department of Health Studies</td><td colspan="2">PATIENT'S NAME</td></tr>
<tr><td>HOSPITAL</td><td>HOSPITAL NUMBER</td></tr>
<tr><td colspan="2">PHYSIOTHERAPY ASSESSMENT
CONTINUATION SHEET</td><td colspan="2">STUDENT PHYSIOTHERAPIST</td></tr>
<tr><td rowspan="2">DATE</td><td colspan="3"><u>PRINCIPLES OF TREATMENT</u>
Aims:

Short-term Goal:

Long-term Goal:

Possible means of achieving aims:

Actual means selected and reasons for choice:

Immediate treatment:

Patient's goal:</td></tr>
<tr><td colspan="3">STAFF COMMENT

CLINICAL SUPERVISOR/LECTURER</td></tr>
</table>

Source: Orientated Record Form.

students use a less detailed form. Similarly, the format can be rearranged to conform to the method of storage used in individual departments or modified to create computerised files.

Essentially, this type of record is centred on the patient's signs and symptoms in order that the student gathers adequate information from which she can identify the patient's main problems. Source-orientated records have been written for specialties also; for example, the Rivermead assessment of motor function in stroke patients (Lincoln and Leadbitter, 1979) and the assessment of upper limb function used at the Hospital for Sick Children, Great Ormond Street (1983).

Visual Displays

Graphic codes and displays may be used so that the progress a patient makes has visual impact. The patient's relative stage of recovery should be immediately apparent and each item of assessment should be displayed in a way that makes more detailed information readily accessible to anyone who needs it. As such a record may be referred to by a wide variety of people, each of them should be able to retrieve accurate and unequivocal information swiftly and easily.

Invented alphabets such as Morse Code and 'sign symptoms' such as those used to direct traffic have been called 'codes for conveying meaning'. An invented alphabet can convey as wide a range of meaning as languages with a traditional alphabet, and a sign system serves a particular purpose in circumstances which rule out the use of alphabets. In either case, conveyance of correct meaning cannot be guaranteed, so selection of either of these alternative ways of communicating information must be based on consideration of the cognitive processing required to comprehend them (Wright, 1981). In order to obviate some misunderstanding, text and graphic codes, such as pictographs and signs, have been juxtaposed on records (see Ashburn, 1982).

Chinese ideograms and musical notation are sign systems which may be considered more successful than traditional alphabets because they can be read and comprehended by people who cannot understand each other's spoken language. Benesh Movement Notation (McGuiness-Scott, 1981/2) is a clinical example of a sign system which transcends spoken language. It is adapted from Benesh Notation used to record the choreography of ballet (Benesh and Benesh, 1977); and it can be used to record gait and other patterns of movement. A stave recording a hemiplegic person's gait is reproduced in Figure 8.2. The transcription below the stave shows that a great deal of information can be conveyed concisely and precisely. Unfortunately, Benesh Movement Notation has

Figure 8.2: An Example of Hemiplegic Gait Written in Benesh Movement Notation

Right hemiplegic gait

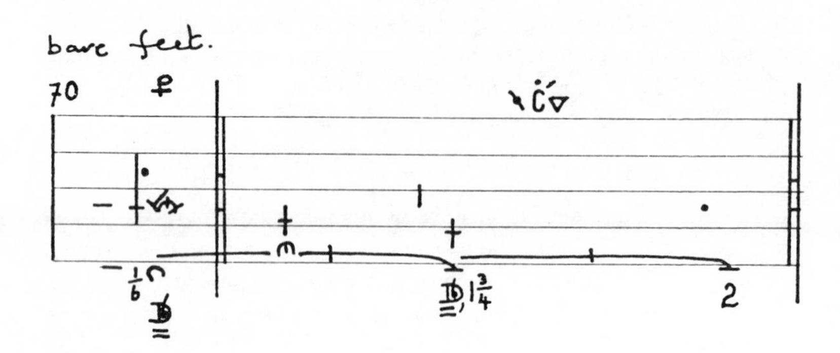

Transcript
STARTING POSTURE (before bar):
Right hip slightly flexed and right shoulder retracted; these two factors are retained throughout the gait.
Right upper limb: elbow flexed; wrist flexed and radially deviated; fingers clenched; hand touching front of body.
Right lower limb: internally rotated; slight plantarflexion; heel just off ground.
Left upper limb: hanging by side.
Left lower limb: in normal position.
Weight-bearing: through both feet; feet slightly apart.
GAIT:
Speed: 70 steps per minute in bare feet; right a quarter short of left.
Right lower limb, swing phase: foot clears ground with ankle plantarflexed; toes stroke ground first.
Right lower limb, stance phase: Heel moves towards ground but does not bear weight; knee flexed until one third of the way through swing of left lower limb, jerks into extension.
Upper limbs: left upper limb swings in normal reciprocal pattern; right upper limb held in starting position.
Left lower limb: normal swing and stance phases.

By courtesy of J. McGuiness-Scott.

limited application because it requires a great deal of learning. Few physiotherapists and even fewer members of other health care professions are trained to use it, so it does not offer a means of communication between physiotherapists at present, let alone a means of interdisciplinary communication.

Precise definition has also been achieved by simpler graphic codes. At the simplest level, directional arrows are very effective. Simple descriptive signs are used by lay people and practitioners involved in the Riding for the Disabled Scheme also. At a more complex level, a sign system for assessment and recording of common problems of vertebral joints is used by physiotherapists internationally (Maitland, 1979; Grieve, 1981).

A sign system has the advantage of conveying a large amount of information in a small space, such as an assessment chart printed on a single sheet. Such a chart needs to accommodate the occasional user, who might refer to it for information 'at a glance' as well as the assessor who uses it regularly. Wright (1970) and Easterby and Hakiel (1981) have shown that an individual's experience and familiarity with specific signs, or with similar signs, influence the likelihood of correct comprehension. Physiotherapists will be more familiar with the item of assessment specified by a particular sign than are other practitioners who refer to the display. They will also learn them more quickly because they use them frequently to administer an assessment and to record their findings as well as to retrieve information. Additionally, signs may be incomprehensible to elderly patients because they have less experience with signs than younger people.

There are few published evaluations of the effectiveness of different types of visual information, but what is known is illustrated by the Sheffield Motor Assessment Chart (Parry, 1982). Following the conventions laid down by Taylor (1971) and Easterby and Hakiel (1977; 1981), correct meaning may be conveyed to different users in different graphic forms:

(1) Information which may be used by patients is presented as written statements; that is, items recording activities such as walking from place to place (Activity Capability).
(2) Information which is utilisable by all members of the rehabilitation team is presented as a system of pictographs or image-related signs which are related to the subject in a particular setting, such as transferring from bed to chair or climbing stairs (Functional Ability and Upper Limb).
(3) Information about the quality of the patient's movement, which has uniquely physiotherapeutic significance and which cannot be represented by a clear image, is represented by numbers or arbitrary signs. They have no visual reference but can be readily learned from the handbook by a physiotherapist (Quality of Movement).

Figure 8.3: Graphic Display

SMAC*

A Physiotherapeutic Assessment of Hemiplegic Patients

Hospital/Unit ____________

Referring Doctor ____________

Physiotherapist

OP/IP **Ward** ____________

AFFIX ADDRESSOGRAPH LABEL

Name ____________

Address ____________

Hospital No. ____________ Age/D. of B. ____________

Date of Onset

Admission Date ____________

Left	Right

Hemiplegia

Left	Right

Handed

Quality of Movement	
14	
13	
12	
11	
10	
9	
8	
7	
6	
5	
4	
3	
2	
1	

Functional Ability in test situation

Activity Capability in non-test situation

		With help of person	▼	▽	Home visit
Can walk safely:	Over slope/ ramp				
	Down flight of stairs				
	Up flight of stairs				
	& negotiate step/kerb				
	To/from lavatory				
	Bedroom to/ from dayroom				
Can get out of/into bed safely					
Can stand up/sit down safely					
Can sit safely on bed-side, lavatory, chair etc.					

Upper Limb

Early Indoor Goal

▼	With support of furniture or walking aid
▽	Totally independently

	To **affected** side		With help of person
	To **unaffected** side		Home visit

Physiotherapy begun: ____________

Dates of assessments:

1 ____________

2 ____________

3 ____________

4 ____________

5 ____________

* The Sheffield Motor Assessment Chart and Handbook are available from: Dr A. Parry, Department of Health Studies, Sheffield City Polytechnic, Collegiate Crescent, Sheffield S10 2BP

Problem Orientated Medical Records

Problem orientated medical records (POMR) were introduced in 1968 by Dr Lawrence Weed of the University of Vermont as a means of recording information about patients' problems and ensuing intervention in a logical format. The method is problem-centred rather than source-centred, as the title indicates, and its format facilitates the retrieval of information. Information is organised under four main headings: data base; problem list; initial plan; and progress notes.

Data base. All relevant subjective and objective information is recorded here, including the patient's personal details, his medical and social histories, and results of the objective examination.

Problem list. This is a comprehensive list of the patient's problems built up from information recorded in the data base. Other relevant conditions and symptoms may be recorded as well as diagnoses. Each problem is numbered, the date on which it was first noticed is recorded and any future reference to a problem is prefixed by its number. By the simple means of placing current problems on an 'active' list and those which have been resolved on an 'inactive' list, resolution of an active problem is recorded by stating the date and indicating by an arrow from it to the inactive list. An explanatory statement may be inserted alongside the problem in the inactive list if necessary. The reverse manoeuvre indicates an inactive problem becoming active. It can be seen from Table 8.3 that the patient's current condition can be appreciated at a glance.

Table 8.3: POMR Problem List

Problem Number	Active	Date	Inactive	Date
1	OA left hip	12.2.83	Arthroplasty	14.2.83
2	Chronic bronchitis	12.2.83		
3	Poor housing	12.2.83	Rehoused	3.9.83
4	Poor mobility following arthroplasty	19.2.83	Walking with gutter frame	1.3.83

Initial plan. A programme of total care for a patient is planned with reference to the problem list. The plan may include the intervention of various practitioners and include diagnostic procedures, surgery, drug therapy, and so on. Similarly, a physiotherapeutic plan can be produced for each appropriate problem, with aims and means referring to the relevant problem number. Methods of treatment and the frequency and duration for which they were applied are recorded also.

Figure 8.4: Problem-orientated Record Sheet

DATA BASE

Surname	No	PT. ....
First Name..........	Date of Birth	OT ....
Address.............	Tel. no.	ST. ....
....		SW ....
Ward		GP ....
Hospital Transport Yes/No		Consultants ......

	Other services involved..............
Occupation	....
Employer	....
School/College	
Hobbies/Interests	Social history ....
....	....
....	....
	Accommodation ....
Benefits	Permanent aids ....
....	....
Claims Pending	....
Past medical history	Communication defect..............
....	....

PHYSIOTHERAPY ASSESSMENT:

Figure 8.4 (contd.)

PROBLEM LIST

Problem no.	Date	Active problem	Date	Inactive problem
1				
2				
3				
4				

INITIAL PLAN

PROGRESS NOTES

SIGNATURE OF PHYSIOTHERAPIST

Table 8.4: SOAP Notes

S:	Subjective note recording what the patient says about his current problems.
O:	Objective note recording findings of repetitions of the objective examination; for example, ROM and tenderness.
A:	Assessment note recording a brief statement of the physiotherapists' interpretation of the current situation and her current goals.
P:	Plan reflecting the outcome of assessments and recording modifications or changes in the original programme, including formulation of new aims.

Progress notes. These can be recorded as a flow chart or, more commonly, as narrative notes. Flow charts are suitable where there are many interrelated problems which are changing over a period of time. The TPR chart is an example. The visual display facilitates understanding and interpretation of data and the frequency of measurement can be varied according to requirements. Narrative notes are written under four headings: subjective; objective; assessment; and plan. The acronym formed by these initials has led to them being referred to as SOAP notes.

Many physiotherapists have found POMR to be a useful method of recording patients' problems and the steps taken to relieve them because its format makes it easier to understand the analytical process underlying the planning of a treatment programme. It also lends itself to simple abstraction of data for research or audit. Its beneficial effect is even more apparent when it is used by all of the practitioners involved in a patient's care.

Summary

No one method of recording is likely to be acceptable to all physiotherapists, however flexible it appears to be. This is particularly so for physiotherapists in specialties who have very specific requirements. Whatever method an individual prefers, general records are required within a department so that data can be put to the types of uses described in Table 8.1.

Adequate and efficient records are vitally important. They provide a clear channel of information; and the logical and analytical approaches to patient care required to produce them improve the quality of practice. Furthermore, they provide a means by which the profession can critically assess techniques and standards of performance. Well presented records supply data for forward planning not only for the physiotherapy service but also for total health care; and the wealth of data stored in patient records can be an invaluable foundation for clinical research. Amongst the plethora of uses it must not be forgotten that, as clinically responsible practitioners, physiotherapists are duty bound to record their activities to meet legal, ethical and professional requirements.

9 GUIDES TO ASSESSMENT

In contrast to the previous section, these Guides are examples of routines for assessing patients with specific conditions or in particular situations. To encourage the learner to develop a systematic approach to investigation, they are presented in a strict sequence: *listen*; *look*; *feel*; *test*; *interpret*.

Assessments of patients with conditions or dysfunctions other than those given here can be based on the same routine, remembering that comprehensive assessment requires a good grasp of the clinical features of a condition and may require examination of several systems. For example, patients with rheumatoid arthritis are commonly referred with 'loss of function' which may be exacerbated by neurological impairment or cardiovascular symptoms.

The unconscious patient presents special problems, especially if he is being ventilated mechanically. Obviously, the patient cannot co-operate and it may be difficult to position him in the optimum position for observations and palpations. Consequently, alternative ways must be found, for example, to assess resonance of the chest. Rate and pattern of breathing cannot be used as indices of disease if breathing is controlled by a ventilator, and it is not possible to palpate the chest where drainage tubes, central venuous pressure lines and incisions are covered by dressings. However, supine position and mechanical ventilation do ease assessment of some items of examination. In particular, the amount of inspired air does not vary and discrepancies between movements on both sides of the chest are immediately apparent.

Guides to assessment of the patient undergoing general surgery and the patient with a musculo-skeletal disorder are given first because they are relatively straightforward and because many students begin their clinical practice on general surgical wards or in out-patient departments. It is expected that, if they are available, medical notes will be read before an assessment is begun and that any student or inexperienced physiotherapist using the Guides will be able to conduct the assessment and to interpret the findings in discussion with an experienced clinician or teacher.

Assessment of the Patient Undergoing General Surgery

Subjective Assessment

(1) History of Present Complaint

Details of *onset*: date and mode; symptoms; course of condition.
List admission — reason for first visit to family doctor; treatment; benefit?
Main problem: influencing factors; changes.
Drugs used: patent or prescribed? benefit derived?

(2) Social History

Occupation: nature of work; what it entails.
Accommodation: flat/house/bungalow? alone/family/others?
Recreational activities.
social habits — *tobacco*/alcohol: amount?

(3) History of Previous Medical Condition

Existing symptoms/dysfunction with bearing on current condition.
Previous *physiotherapy*? outcome?

Objective Assessment

(1) General Observation

TPR — read chart, note values.
Appearance: posture, build, colour; position in bed; comfortable, distressed, in pain?

(2) Local Observation

Shape of chest.
Respiration: rate, depth, level, pattern; wheezing?
Cough: type, frequency, severity.
Sputum: amount, character, viscosity.
Haemoptysis: type, amount.
Chest pain: type, location.

(3) Palpation

Breathing: localisation and bilateral equality.
Resonance of chest sounds.
Calf, if complaint of tenderness (DVT).

(4) Tests and Measurements in case of post-operative complications

Auscultation: breath sounds heard? vesicular or bronchial? adventitious sounds?
Radiographs: translucency of lung fields; identification of segments for postural drainage.

(5) Medical Data

Read admission notes pre-operatively.
Read operation notes.

Interpretation

List of problems in priority order.
Aims of treatment, with direct relevance to assessment and list of problems.
Means: possible means of achieving aims; actual means selected; reasons for choice.
Plan of treatment.
Reassessments: record progress; reassess regularly; modify as necessary.

Assessment of the Patient with a Peripheral Musculo-skeletal Disorder

Subjective Assessment

(1) History of Present Complaint

Reason treatment sought: pain, stiffness, instability/giving way, weakness, loss of function; trauma, fracture, dislocation, etc.
Details of *onset*: *injury* — date and mode, symptoms, location and extent of immediate pain, course of condition; *spontaneous* — location, predisposing and influencing factors, progress.
Symptoms and location: record large joints on body chart.
Visit to family doctor: treatment; benefit?
Drugs used: patent or prescribed? benefit derived?

(2) Social History

Occupation: nature of work; what it entails.
Accommodation: flat/house/bungalow? alone/family/others?
Recreational activities.

(3) History of Previous Medical Condition

Existing symptoms/dysfunction with bearing on current condition.
Previous *physiotherapy*? outcome?

Objective Assessment

(1) General Observation

Appearance: posture, build, colour; comfortable, distressed, in pain?
Movement: willingness to move part; patterns.
Gait.
Orthopaedic appliances.

(2) Local Observation

Skin: colour and condition.
Contour and alignment: muscle wasting, swelling, effusion, deformity.

(3) Palpation

Skin: texture; temperature of area.
Soft tissues: thickening, tenderness/pain/hypersensitivity — focal/referred.
Swelling: type and feel.
Muscular tone: normal/flabby/spasm.
Movements: passive; accessory.

(4) Tests and Measurements

Muscle power.
Muscle bulk.
Stability and integrity of joints.
Range of movement/fixed deformities/length of lower limbs.

(5) Medical Data

Read medical notes.
Read reports of radiographs.
Read reports of medical laboratory tests.

Interpretation

List of problems in priority order.
Aims of treatment, with direct relevance to assessment and list of problems. Short-term goal(s); long-term goal(s).
Means: possible means of achieving aims; actual means selected; reasons for choice.
Plan of treatment.
Reassessments: record progress; reassess regularly; modify as necessary.

Assessment of the Patient with a Disorder of the Back

Subjective Assessment

(1) History of Present Complaint

Reason treatment sought: pain, stiffness, weakness, loss of function.
Details of *onset*: *injury* — date and mode, course of condition; *insidious* — location, predisposing and influencing factors, progress.
Symptoms and location (record on body chart).
Pain: constant — varying in intensity, influencing factors; *inconstant* — predisposing factors.
Visit to family doctor: treatment; benefit?
Drugs used: patent or prescribed? benefit derived?

(2) Social History

Occupation: nature of work; what it entails.
Accommodation: flat/house/bungalow? alone/family/others?
Recreational activities.

(3) History of Previous Medical Condition

Existing symptoms/dysfunction with bearing on current condition: frequency of occurrence, duration, relief.
Previous *physiotherapy*? outcome?

Objective Assessment of muscles and joints under symptomatic area and of joints which may refer symptoms.

(1) General Observation

Appearance: build, colour; comfortable, distressed, in pain?
Posture: in lying, sitting and standing.
Movement: willingness to move; patterns of movement.
Gait.
Orthopaedic appliances.

(2) Local Observation

Skin: colour and condition.
Contour and alignment: muscle wasting, swelling, effusion.
Deformity: scoliosis/kyphosis.

(3) Palpation

Skin: texture; temperature of area.
Soft tissues: thickening; tenderness/pain/hypersensitivity — focal/referred.
Swelling: type and feel.
Muscular tone: local or extensive spasm; inhibited.
Movements: passive; accessory.

(4) Tests and Measurements

Magnitude of tendon reflexes.
Power and action of muscles: myotomes (isometric contraction).
Range of movement/fixed deformities/length of lower limbs.
Sensation: cutaneous appreciation; dermatomes (on body chart).
Spinal tests: passive straight leg raise, passive neck flexion, etc.

(5) Medical Data

Reports of radiographs.

Interpretation

List of problems in priority order.
Aims of treatment, with direct relevance to assessment and list of problems. Short-term goal(s); long-term goal(s).
Means: possible means of achieving aims; actual means selected; reasons for choice.
Plan of treatment.
Reassessments: record progress; reassess regularly; modify as necessary.

Assessment of the Patient with Chronic Obstructive Airways Disease

Subjective Assessment

(1) History of Present Complaint

Details of *mode of onset*: symptoms; course of condition.
Main reason for first visit to family doctor: treatment; benefit?
Main problem: influencing factors; changes.
Estimate of own *functional capacity*.
Drugs used: patent or prescribed? benefit derived?

(2) Social History

Occupation: nature of work; what it entails.
Change in last 5 years? reason? intention to change now?
Accommodation: flat/house/bungalow? alone/family/others?
Recreational activities.
Change in life-style due to condition?

(3) History of Previous Medical Condition

Existing symptoms/dysfunction with bearing on current condition.
Previous *physiotherapy*? outcome?

Objective Assessment

(1) General Observation

Appearance: posture, build, colour; comfortable, distressed, in pain?

(2) Local Observation

Shape of chest.
Respiration: rate, depth, level, pattern.
Cough: type, frequency, severity.
Sputum: amount, character, viscosity.
Haemoptysis: type, amount.
Chest pain: type, location.
Signs of cardiorespiratory insufficieny: dyspnoea; orthopnoea; ankle and sacral oedema; raised JVP; cyanosis.

(3) Palpation

Breathing: localisation and bilateral equality.
Resonance of chest sounds.
Fremitus.

(4) Tests and Measurements

Chest measurements.
Auscultation: breath sounds heard? vesicular or bronchial? adventitious sounds?
Radiographs: translucency of lung fields; cardiac shadow.
Lung function tests: FVC, FEV_1, PEFR.
Exercise tolerance related to functional ability.

(5) Medical Data

Analyses of blood gases.

Interpretation

List of problems in priority order.
Aims of treatment, with direct relevance to assessment and list of problems. Short-term goal(s); long-term goal(s).
Means: possible means of achieving aims; actual means selected; reasons for choice.
Plan of treatment.
Reassessments: record progress; reassess regularly; modify as necessary.

Assessment of the Mechanically Ventilated Patient in a Cardiothoracic or Neurosurgical Intensive Care Unit

Subjective Assessment from medical notes of unconscious patient

(1) History of Present Complaint

Details of *onset*: date; mode — injury/elective surgery/medical condition; signs; course of condition.

(2) Social History

Occupation: nature of work; what it entails.
Accommodation: flat/house/bungalow? alone/family/others?

(3) History of Previous Medical Condition

Existing symptoms/dysfunction with bearing on current condition.
Previous *physiotherapy*? outcome?

Objective Assessment (Inspection in Supine)

(1) General Observation

Temperature and pulse: read chart, note values.
Appearance: posture, build, colour; comfortable, distressed, in pain? moving? patterns of movement.
Restrictions on examination: evidence of trauma; previous incisions; dressings on tubes, CVP lines, incisions.

(2) Local Observation

Skin: condition; subcutaneous emphysema.
Shape of chest: anteroposterior diameter; kyphoscoliosis.
Bilateral equality of chest movement (NB tubes and lines).
Sputum: amount; character; viscosity.
Haemoptysis: frank/stained/streaky/rusty.
Drainage tubes: blood in tube? functioning correctly?
Signs of cardiopulmonary insufficiency: oedema; JVP; cyanosis.

(3) Palpation

Ventilation of lobes (NB tubes, lines and dressings).
Fremitus: rhonchi; transmitted from airways?
Crepitus due to fractured ribs?
Resonance: percussion over anterior chest wall.
Muscular tone: normal/hypotonic/spastic/spasm.

(4) Tests and Measurements

Auscultation: breath sounds heard? vesicular or bronchial? adventitious sounds?
Chest radiographs: translucency of lung fields; cardiac shadow; abnormalities; identification of segments for postural drainage.

(5) Medical Data

Air bronchograms if performed.
Analyses of blood gases.
Readings available from monitoring devices, e.g. thoracic/lung compliance from airway pressure gauge of ventilator; intracranial pressure of patient with head injury.

Interpretation

List of problems in priority order.
Aims of treatment, with direct relevance to assessment and list of problems. Short-term goal(s); long-term goal(s).
Means: possible means of achieving aims; actual means selected; reasons for choice.
Plan of treatment.
Reassessments: record progress; reassess regularly; modify as necessary.

Assessment of a Patient with a Peripheral Nerve Injury

Subjective Assessment

(1) History of Present Complaint

Details of *mode of onset*: symptoms; course of condition.
Main problem: influencing factors? extent? changes?
Treatment already received? type? from whom? effect?
Drugs used: patent or prescribed? benefit derived?

(2) Social History

Occupation: nature of work; what it entails; ability to cope? intention to change?
Accommodation: flat/house/bungalow? alone/family/others?
Recreational activities.
Change in life-style due to condition?

(3) History of Previous Medical Condition

Existing symptoms/dysfunction with bearing on condition.
Previous *physiotherapy*? outcome?

Objective Assessment

(1) General Observation

Appearance.
Attitudes of limb: flaccid; contractures and deformities; aids and appliances.
Movements: trick movements, functional movement.

(2) Local Observation

Skin: colour, condition, nails.
Contours: swelling, muscle wasting.

(3) Palpation

Skin: texture; temperature of area related to ambient temperature.
Soft tissues: extensibility; mobility; tenderness/hypersensitivity.
Swelling: type; feel.
Muscular tone: normal/flabby.
Movements: passive; accessory.

(4) Tests and Measurements

Magnitude of tendon reflexes.
Power and action of individual muscles.
Muscle bulk.
Range of movement: active, passive; accessory movements.
Electrical reactions.
Sensory appreciation — record on body chart.

(5) Medical Data

Electromyography and nerve conduction studies.

Interpretation

List of problems in priority order.
Aims of treatment, with direct relevance to assessment and list of problems. Short-term goal(s); long-term goal(s) with realistic approach to prognosis.
Means: taking account of patient's age and life-style.
Plan of treatment.
Reassessments: record progress; reassess regularly; modify.

Assessment of the Patient with Rheumatoid Arthritis

Subjective Assessment

(1) History of Present Complaint

Details of *onset*: mode — insidious or acute; date; symptoms — pain and stiffness of single joints/multiple joints; rate and pattern of progression.
Each joint involved: mildly/severely; acute/subacute/chronic.
Main problems: pain, stiffness, instability/giving way, weakness, loss of function.
Functional activities: description of disability.
Systemic manifestations: generalised sweating; dry eyes, dry mouth and difficulty swallowing (Sjogren's syndrome); SOBOE (cardiovascular involvement); incontinence.
Treatment received: from whom? benefit?
Drugs used: patent or prescribed? benefit derived?

(2) Social History

Occupation: nature of work; what it entails.
Change during last 5 years? reason? intention to change now?
Accommodation: flat/house/bungalow? alone/family/others?
aids and adaptations? need to move?
Recreational activities.
Change in life-style due to condition?

(3) History of Previous Medical Condition

Existing symptoms/dysfunction with bearing on current condition.
Previous *physiotherapy*? outcome?

Objective Assessment

(1) General Observation

Appearance: posture, build, colour; comfortable, distressed, in pain?
Distribution of joints involved: feet, hands and wrists; knees, hips; elbows, shoulders; cervical spine.
Movement: willingness to move; patterns of movement.
Gait: due to pain and stiffness/foot drop/spastic paraplegia.
Orthopaedic appliances.

(2) Local Observation

Skin: atrophied, friable; vasculitic lesions.
Contour: muscle wasting, swelling, effusion, nodules.
Subcutaneous masses on pressure areas: elbows, sacrum, tendo achilles, other tendons.
Deformity of joints: swan neck; subluxation of MTP joints ('walking on marbles'); disruption of other joints.

(3) Palpation

Skin: texture; tenderness.
Joints: swelling; temperature; pain on movement.
Soft tissues: tenderness and pain; thickenings, nodules, mobility, extensibility.

(4) Tests and Measurements

Power and action of muscles.
Stability and integrity of joints.
Range of movement: active and passive range of affected and unaffected joints; accessory movements; fixed deformities.
Motor and sensory for signs of: compression neuropathies; peripheral neuropathy; compression of cervical cord.
Functional ability.
Chest radiographs: pleural effusion; pulmonary fibrosis; pericardial effusion.
Radiographs of joints: loss of space; erosion of bone; secondary osteoarthrosis.

(5) Medical Data

Reports of biopsy of synovial membrane and microbiological examination of synovial fluid.

Interpretation

List of problems in priority order.
Aims of treatment, with direct relevance to assessment and list of problems. Short-term goal(s); long-term goal(s).
Means: possible means of achieving aims; actual means selected; reasons for choice.
Plan of treatment.
Reassessments: record progress; reassess regularly; modify as necessary.

Assessment of the Patient with a Neurological Condition

Subjective Assessment

(1) History of Present Complaint

Details of *mode of onset*: symptoms; course of condition.
Understanding of condition.
Family doctor visited? why? treatment? benefit?
Drugs used: patent or prescribed? benefit derived?

(2) Social History

Occupation: employed? nature of work; what it entails.
Change in last 5 years? reason? need to change now?
Accommodation: flat/house/bungalow? alone/family/others?
Recreational activities?
Estimate of own functional capacity.
Potential effect of condition on life-style?

(3) History of Previous Medical Condition

Existing symptoms/dysfunction with bearing on condition.
Previous *physiotherapy*? outcome?

Objective Assessment

(1) Observation and Palpation

Relative age: chronological age compared with apparent age.
Attitude: co-operative/indifferent/enthusiastic/aggressive; euphoric/depressive/labile/normal.
Orientation: time and space.
Communication: normal/dysarthric/dysphasic/aphrasic; hearing; concrete matters, abstract matters; reading, writing, numeracy.
Posture in supine, sitting and standing; symmetry; alignment of head, trunk and limb girdles; attitudes of limbs.
Muscle tone: flaccidity/hypotonia/spasticity/rigidity.
Quality of movement: patterns of movement; influence of reflex activity; involuntary movement; bradykinesia/akinesia.
Gait.
Functional activities: mobility, dressing, grooming, feeding, etc.
Dexterity: large objects; small objects; fine movements.

(2) Tests and Measurements

Magnitude of tendon reflexes.
Pathological synergies.
Automatic postural adjustment/balance reactions.
Sensory appreciation, perception and cognition: cutaneous and proprioceptive input; co-ordination; integration and perception; visual fields.

Interpretation

List of problems in priority order.
Aims of treatment, with direct relevance to assessment and list of problems. Short-term goal(s) and long-term goal(s) with realistic approach to prognosis.
Means: taking account of patient's age and life-style.
Plan of treatment.
Reassessments: record progress; reassess regularly; modify.

Assessment of the Stroke Patient

Subjective Assessment

(1) History of Present Complaint

Details of *mode of onset*: symptoms; course of condition.
Understanding of condition.
Family doctor visited? why? treatment? benefit?
Drugs used: patent or prescribed? benefit derived?

(2) Social History

Occupation: nature of work; what it entails.
Change in last 5 years? reason? need to change now?
Accommodation: flat/house/bungalow? alone/family/others?
Recreational activities?
Potential effect of stroke on life-style?

(3) History of Previous Medical Condition

Existing symptoms/dysfunction with bearing on condition.
Previous *physiotherapy*? outcome?

Objective Assessment

(1) Observation and Palpation

(a) Appearance
Relative age: chronological age compared with apparent age.
Attitude: co-operative/indifferent/enthusiastic/aggressive; euphoric/depressed/labile/normal.
Orientation: time and space.
Communication: normal/dysarthric/dysphasic/aphrasic; concrete matters, abstract matters; reading, writing, numeracy.
(b) Early patient
Posture in supine: symmetry; alignment of head, trunk and limb girdles; attitudes of limbs.
Muscle tone: flaccidity/hypotonia/hypertonia.
Quality of movement: patterns of movement; influence of reflex activity.

(c) Recovering patient
Posture in sitting and standing.
Muscle tone.
Quality of movement: patterns of movement; rolling in bed, getting out of bed, etc.
Gait.
Functional activities: mobility, dressing, grooming, feeding, etc.

(2) Tests and Measurements

Magnitude of tendon reflexes.
Pathological synergies.
Automatic postural adjustment/balance reactions.
Sensory appreciation, perception and cognition: cutaneous and proprioceptive input; integration and perception; visual fields.

Interpretation

List of problems in priority order.
Aims of treatment, with direct relevance to assessment and list of problems. Short-term goal(s) and long-term goal(s) with realistic approach to prognosis.
Means: taking account of patient's age and life-style.
Plan of treatment.
Reassessments: record progress; reassess regularly; modify.

REFERENCES AND RECOMMENDED READING

Acheson, R. M. and Hall, D. J. (1976) Epilogue in R. M. Acheson, D. J. Hall, and L. Aird (eds.), *Seminars in Community Medicine, Volume 2: Health Information, Planning and Monitoring*, Oxford University Press, London

Argyle, M. (1972) *The Psychology of Interpersonal Behaviour*, Penguin Books, Harmondsworth

——— (ed.) (1981) *Social Skills and Health*, Methuen, London and New York

Ashburn, A. (1982) 'A Physical Assessment for Stroke Patients', *Physiotherapy, 68* (4), 109–13

Baer, E., Davitz, L. J. and Lieb, R. (1970) 'Inferences of Physical Pain and Psychological Distress: 1. In Relation to Verbal and Non-verbal Patient Communication', *Nursing Research, 19* (5), 388–91

Belcher, J. R. and Sturridge, M. F. (1972) *Thoracic Surgical Management*, Bailliere Tindall, London

Benesh, R. and Benesh, J. (1977) *The Birth of Choreology*, Souvenir Press, London

Bernstein, L., Bernstein, R. S. and Dana, R. H. (1974) *Interviewing: A Guide for Health Professionals*, Appleton-Century-Crofts, New York

Bowsher, D. (1978) *Mechanisms of Nervous Disorder: An Introduction*, Blackwell Scientific, Oxford

Bromley, A. I. (1978) 'The Patient Care Audit', *Physiotherapy, 64* (9)

——— (1983) 'Facts and Fantasies', *Physiotherapy, 69* (11), 384–9

Carr, J. H. and Shepherd, R. (1980) *Physiotherapy in Disorders of the Brain*, William Heinemann Medical Books, London

Cochrane, A. L. (1972) *Effectiveness and Efficiency*, Nuffield Provincial Hospitals Trust, London

Cook, M. (1979) *Perceiving Others*, Methuen, London and New York

Critchley, M. (1953) *The Parietal Lobes*, Hafner, New York

Crofton, J. and Douglas, A. (1969) *Respiratory Diseases*, Blackwell Scientific, Oxford

Cross, H. D. (1974) 'The Case for Problem Orientated Medical Records'., *British Journal of Hospital Medicine, 11*, 65–79

Department of Health and Social Security (1973) *The Remedial Professions* (McMillan Report), Her Majesty's Stationery Office, London

——— Welsh Office (1972) *Rehabilitation: Report of a Subcommittee of the Standing Medical Advisory Committee* (Tunbridge Report), Her Majesty's Stationery Office, London

Easterby, R. S. and Hakiel, S. R. (1977) *Safety Labelling of Consumer Products: Shape and Colour Code Stereotypes in the Design of Signs*, AP Report 75, University of Aston in Birmingham

———, ——— (1981) 'Field Testing of Consumer Safety Signs: The Comprehension of Pictorially Presented Messages', *Applied Ergonomics, 12* (3), 143–52

Enelow, A. J. and Swisher, S. N. (1972) *Interviewing and Patient Care*, Oxford University Press, New York

Evans, D. M. D. (1978) *Special Tests and their Meanings*, Faber, London and Boston

Fowler, H. W. (1926) *A Dictionary of Modern English Usage*, Oxford University Press, London

Franklin, S., Perry, A. and Beatty, A. (1983) *Living with Parkinson's Disease*, The Parkinson's Disease Society, London

French, R. M. (1975) *Guide to Diagnostic Procedures*, McGraw-Hill, New York

Froelich, R. E. and Bishop, F. M. (1977) *Clinical Interviewing Skills: A Programmed Manual for Data Gathering, Evaluation and Patient Managmenet*, C. V. Mosby, St Louis, Missouri

Gagahan, J. (1975) *Interpersonal and Group Behaviour*, Methuen, London and New York

Gowers, E. (1977) *The Complete Plain Words*, rev. edn, Penguin Books, Harmondsworth
Graves, S. (1971) 'Better Records: First Steps to Better Quality. Problem Orientated Record is Key to Better Medical Practice', *Modern Hospital* (116)
Grieve, G. P. (1975) *Mobilisation of the Spine*, Churchill Livingstone, Edinburgh
——— (1981) *Common Vertebral Joint Problems*, Churchill Livingstone, Edinburgh
Heath, J. R. (1978) 'Problem Orientated Medical Systems', *Physiotherapy, 64* (9)
Hospital for Sick Children, Great Ormond Street (1983) *Basic Guidelines for Physiotherapy Assessment*
——— (1983) *Basic Guidelines for Physiotherapy Assessment of Upper Limb Function*
Illich, I. (1975) *Medical Nemesis*, Marion Boyars, London
Lincoln, N. and Leadbitter (1979) 'Assessment of Motor Function in Stroke Patients', *Physiotherapy, 65* (2), 48–51
Loftus, E. F., Freedman, J. L. and Loftus, G. R. (1970) 'Retrieval of Words from Subordinate and Supraordinate Categories in Semantic Hierarchies', *Psychonomic Science* (21), 235–6
Lubbock, G. (1983) *Stroke Care: An Interdisciplinary Approach*, Faber, London and Boston
Luria, A. R. (1975) *The Man with the Shattered World*, Penguin Books, Harmondsworth
McCaffery, M. (1983) *Nursing the Patient in Pain*, Harper and Row, London
McGuiness-Scott, J. (1981/2) 'Benesh Movement Notation', *Physiotherapy, 67/8*
McIntyre, N. and Petrie, J. C. (1979) *The Problem Orientated Medical Record*, Churchill Livingstone, London
Mackenzie, C. F., Ciesla, N., Imle, P. C. and Klemic, N. (1981) *Chest Physiotherapy in the Intensive Care Unit*, Williams and Wilkins, Baltimore and London
McRae, R. (1976) *Clinical Orthopaedic Examination*, Churchill Livingstone, Edinburgh
Maitland, G. D. (1979) *Musculo-skeletal Examination and Recording Guide*, Lauderdale Press, Glen Osmond, South Australia
Medical Research Council (1943) *War Memorandum No. 7: Investigation of Peripheral Nerve Injuries*, Her Majesty's Stationery Office, London
Melzack, R. and Wall, P. W. (1982) *The Challenge of Pain*, Penguin Books, Harmondsworth
National Health Service (1977) circular HC(77)33, Department of Health and Social Security, London
Panayi, G. S. (1980) *Essential Rheumatology for Nurses and Therapists*, Bailliere Tindall, London
Parry, A. W. (1982) 'Development and Evaluation of the Sheffield Motor Assessment Chart', unpublished PhD thesis, CNAA; assessment folder reprinted (1984) by CIBA Laboratories
Partridge, C. J. (1980) 'The Effectiveness of Physiotherapy: A Classification for Evaluation', *Physiotherapy, 66* (5), 153–5
Partridge, E. (1957) *Usage and Abusage: A Guide to Good English*, Penguin Books, Harmondsworth
Professions Supplementary to Medicine Act (1960) 8 & 9 Eliz. 2 c. 66
Sachs, O. W. (1976) *Awakenings*, Random House, New York and London
Shepherd, R. (1974) *Physiotherapy in Paediatrics*, William Heinemann Medical Books, London
Spence, J. C. (1953) 'Methodology of Clinical Science', *Lancet* (2), 629
Stickland, A. (1984) 'Examination of the Knee Joint', *Physiotherapy, 70* (4), 144–50
Taylor, R. (1971) *A Basic Course in Graphic Design*, Studio Vista, London
Waller, R. H. W. (1979) 'Four Aspects of Graphic Communication', *Instructional Science* (8), 213–22
Weed, L. (1968) 'Medical Records that Guide and Teach', *New England Journal of Medicine, 278*, 593–600, 652–7
——— (1971) 'Quality Control and Medical Records', *Archives of Internal Medicine, 127*, 100–5
Wicksteed, J. H. (1948) *The Growth of a Profession*, Edward Arnold, London

Williams, J. I. (1983) 'The Responsibility for Physiotherapy Prescription', *Physiotherapy, 69* (12), 435

World Health Organization (1980) *International Classification of Impairments, Disabilities and Handicap*, World Health Organization, Geneva

Wright, A. (1970) *Designing for Visual Aids*, Studio Vista London

Wright, P. (1981) ' "The Instructions Clearly State . . . " Can't People Read?', *Applied Ergonomics, 6* (4), 213–20

Zborowski, M. (1969) *People in Pain*, Jossey Bass, San Francisco

Zola, I. K. (1966) 'Culture and Symptoms — An Analysis of Patients Complaining Presenting Complaints', *American Sociological Review, 31* (5), 615–30

INDEX